MORE PRAISE FOR DR. DINUBILE AND *FrameWork*

"NO DOUBT ABOUT IT, *FrameWork* is an important book that I know you will enjoy and find helpful on your road to optimal health, conditioning, and achievement. It's a must-read for anyone who cares about his or her body and wants it to last."

—Governor Arnold Schwarzenegger

"During my 21-year major-league career it was amazing to see the advances in training and medicine from the time I first made it to the big leagues in 1981 to the time I retired in 2001. Dr. DiNubile's book is a striking example of that and how a firm understanding of your body and how best to keep it in shape can enhance every part of your life. Having gone through my share of injuries, from bumps and bruises to a herniated disk, I wish that resources like *FrameWork* were available to me throughout my career."

—Cal Ripken, Jr.,
baseball's all-time "Iron Man," two-time AL MVP, perennial All-Star

"Dr. Nick has the uncanny ability to understand the language of the human body. He knows how it speaks. In the movie industry and in sports, the body is invaluable as an instrument. Dr. Nick is invaluable at keeping that instrument tuned to perfection. He is a healer of the highest order."

—M. Night Shyamalan,
The Sixth Sense, Unbreakable,
The Last Airbender

"*FrameWork* is an indispensable text that gives individuals essential advice and information on how to protect and enhance arguably our most valuable asset—the health and function of our musculoskeletal systems. Renowned orthopedic surgeon Dr. Nicholas DiNubile offers a wide variety of useful tips and practical guidance such as how to conduct a simple self-assessment of the condition of our muscles, bones, and joints, and, more importantly, how to properly exercise to safely improve our functional movement capabilities. At the American Council on Exercise, we were so impressed with the content in *FrameWork* that it is used as the core foundation of a continuing education course for our more than 50,000 fitness professionals. This book is a must-read for anyone interested in experiencing the joys of leading a physically active lifestyle and developing a body that's built to last a lifetime."

—Cedric X. Bryant, PhD, FACSM,
chief science officer, American Council on Exercise

"I have known Dr. DiNubile for many years, and his reputation as a specialist in sports medicine is legendary. Now he has compiled into book form knowledge accumulated from many years of working with athletes, which should enable even the nonathlete to achieve total fitness."

—Kenneth H. Cooper, MD, MPH,
founder, president, and CEO, The Cooper Aerobics Center

"This is the owner's manual that should have come with your body."

—Dr. Neil Liebman,
team chiropractor, Philadelphia 76ers

"Dr. Nick is a great doctor. He's not only an excellent surgeon but also an understanding, feeling practitioner in all musculoskeletal-related concerns. As he says, since we are living longer, this aspect of health care has surpassed the common cold for frequency of treatment. I am fortunate enough to have had Dr. Nick repair one of my knees. Being a good example of just the kind of extended-wear person Dr. Nick is talking about, now I am even more grateful to get advice from one of the brightest (and nicest) guys in the field on how to keep my frame working for me. I, like a lot of us who have borrowed time from science, can only very strongly recommend his words to anyone and everyone interested in keeping their bones working to their best potential as we gracefully glide, run, skip, bat, pole-vault, hike, or bike into our happiest days."

—William Hurt,
Academy Award–winning actor

"Dr. DiNubile is the master of preventative medicine for the musculoskeletal system."

—Wayne L. Westcott, PhD, CSCS,
fitness research director, South Shore YMCA, Quincy, MA

"*FrameWork* teaches you how to take optimal care of your body so you can enjoy both life and leisure more. For athletes, it's essential for a long healthy career."

—Jay Sigel,
U.S. PGA and U.S. amateur golf champion

"Dr. DiNubile's *FrameWork* provides cutting-edge information not only from a health and wellness standpoint but from an athletic performance aspect as well."

—Gary Vitti,
head trainer, LA Lakers

"I was quite young when a knee injury changed my life. Dr. Nick helped me then, and he can help you now."

—David Boreanaz,
actor, *Bones*, *Angel*, and *Buffy the Vampire Slayer*

FrameWork

for the
KNEE

A 6-STEP PLAN FOR PREVENTING
INJURY AND ENDING PAIN

NICHOLAS A. DiNUBILE, MD
with Bruce Scali

RODALE

© 2010 by Nicholas A. DiNubile, MD

Rodale books may be purchased for business or promotional use or for special sales. For information, please write to: Special Markets Department, Rodale Inc., 733 Third Avenue, New York, NY 10017

Printed in the United States of America
Rodale Inc. makes every effort to use acid-free ⊚, recycled paper ♻.
Illustrations by Karen Kuchar
Photographs by Mitch Mandel

Book design by Christina Gaugler

Library of Congress Cataloging-in-Publication Data is on file with the publisher.
DiNubile, Nicholas A.
  Framework for the knee : a 6-step plan for preventing injury and ending pain / Nicholas A. DiNubile ; with Bruce Scali.
    p.   cm.
  Includes index.
  ISBN 978-1-60529-593-0 paperback
  1. Knee—Wounds and injuries—Exercise therapy.   2. Knee—Wounds and injuries—Prevention.   I. Scali, Bruce.   II. Title.
RD561.D65   2010
617.5'82044—dc22   2010032435

Distributed to the trade by Macmillan
    6   8   10   9   7   5   paperback

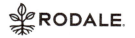

We inspire and enable people to improve their lives and the world around them.

To my dream team:
Marybeth, Emily, and Dylan

CONTENTS

PREFACE

The circumstances couldn't have been better when I started this installment in the series that is dear to me. Two inches of snow were on every twig outside my window in the suburbs of Philadelphia and the Winter Olympics were in full swing, and the knee in all its glory was center stage in the visions that played in my mind's eye of skaters on local ponds, of children frolicking in the snow or swooshing on their sleds, and of the finest athletes in the world doing their thing in Vancouver. The critical importance of our frames' fulcrums for healthy motion—on any day in any venue—was brought into sharp relief, and I was reminded for the zillionth time that getting our bodies to do what we want them to do depends in large measure on hinges that are inherently unsteady.

Fortunately, when Mother Nature put us together, she stabilized our knees and other joints with a couple of critical connective and neural components that, in a perfect world, work together in fine-tuned coordination without us being conscious of it. (This is known as *proprioception*. I know it's a big word, and I promise to keep that kind to a minimum, but it applies to multiple areas of your body and is critical for smooth, controlled, precise motion. And smooth motion is how you extend the warranty on your frame that I'm always talking about.) So you go on your merry way and don't think about your knees at all. Until . . .

You suffer a sports injury like I did, or . . .
Something just isn't right about them, or . . .
One of them goes out on you again, or . . .
Wear and tear breaks down a part or two.
Or three.

Hence the millions of patients of every age who limp or hobble into orthopedic offices seeking relief. And that's right up my alley.

KNEE BENT

In med school I thought I was on my way to becoming a hand surgeon until I fell in love with a wonderful new toy—the arthroscope—that was used solely on the knee at that point in time. Prior to the introduction of that marvelous invention, my surgical training consisted of opening the knee from stem to stern with multiple incisions, taking the knee apart, and trying to put it back together. To be polite, I'll say results were mixed; we had our successes, but too many knees were destroyed in an effort to save them.

They were just starting to use the scope as a surgical (rather than diagnostic only) tool when I was in my residency at Penn. I sure was fortunate to be able to set up my chief year working with two arthroscopy pioneers, Dr. John Joyce and Dr. Jim Nixon, who was one of the Philadelphia Eagles' doctors at the time. These courageous surgeons poked around the knee joint and couldn't always see what they wanted to do (the scopes and accessory instrumentation were pretty primitive then), but they forged ahead.

I was right behind them. I couldn't get enough exposure to the scope, and I was every bit as hooked on its potential as my mentors were. It was my kind of tool—very precise, and it required a minimal incision. It was my first exposure to the concept that one could actually accelerate healing and minimize downtime—something critical for athletes, and quite appealing for just about everyone else.

Speaking of athletes, I believe it was fate that had me working under one of the fathers of sports medicine (also a new and emerging field at the time), Dr. Joe Torg. Dr. Torg took me under his wing, and I began to cover many of the sports teams and events in our region. He was a "kneecentric" doc, and I found my calling in the world of sports medicine, with a primary interest in the knee. My training at the University of Pennsylvania also allowed me to form a lifelong connection and friendship with a world-renowned knee replacement surgeon, Dr. Paul Lotke, whom I joined in private practice after completing my surgical training. I guess I was just destined to be a knee guy.

JOINT DISCUSSION

Midway through my residency, I went to an orthopedic conference out in Utah that offered a pretty well-known arthroscopy course. My buddy Mark and I were looking at the schedule and trying to figure out . . . um, you know how it is—we were young, recreational sports freaks, and we just had to fit in some during our stay. We assured ourselves that we were there to listen a lot and learn a lot, but we thought, *Hey, we're in Salt Lake City and there's no way we're not going to get some skiing in, what with Park City and other resort areas being so nearby.*

Mindful of our second purpose, we pored over the schedule and came upon a guy named Lanny Johnson who was a real pioneer in our field. He was one of those visionaries who are willing to try seemingly crazy futuristic stuff that, frankly, I don't know if we can do anymore because of restraints that shackle physicians these days, especially in the United States, in terms of innovation (something that concerns me quite a bit). Anyway, Lanny would be showing an ACL reconstruction performed through the scope (something no one else was doing at the time), and that wasn't to be missed, either.

Once a guy like Lanny has an idea and breaks it down for others, then over the next 10 years the tools get better, the techniques get better, and it's a lot easier to operate. He was working with existing tools that weren't designed for how he worked with them. My buddy and I were transfixed as we watched Lanny's procedure, how he used big drills we would use for major open surgeries like fractures or for joint replacement. He bored up onto the femur with visibility in the knee akin to skiing or driving in a blizzard, and I remember turning to my friend Mark and saying, "Let's go skiing right now because I can tell you I am never going to try anything like that!" Talk about crazy.

That was around 1982, when arthroscopic surgery was in its infancy and its rank today in the top five most commonly performed procedures was incomprehensible. We were just learning to take out the meniscus, so the idea of doing an ACL reconstruction without opening the knee and drilling all around in there was madness to me. I thought, *Lanny sure is brave, but he's out of his mind for trying something like that, something I will never do.*

Yes, my buddy and I schussed then. But we went back to school on advanced arthroscopy, too, and not too long after Lanny's presentation, I performed the first arthroscopic ACL reconstruction in my region. Thanks to him and other trailblazing mentors of mine, I learned firsthand that it was, indeed, crazy.

Crazy brilliant.

And one of the things I do all the time now.

KNEEPAD

The arthroscope was first used on the knee, but now is placed in a wide variety of joints.

The interesting thing about being a surgeon, and this surely applies to other fields as well, is that I'm not doing anything I was first trained to do during my extensive surgical training. I got a solid foundation and a set of skills early on, served as an apprentice to other surgeons, and watched a lot and tried a little bit under direct supervision, but I also learned that manual skills, the way one thinks, and technology are going to change, so I had to be prepared for progress. Although I was fortunate to begin my career at a time when fantastic innovation was afoot, I know that progress usually isn't about a giant leap as was done with the scope. Each advance adds one skill to the set already being applied, and I know in 10 to 15 years I'll be doing stuff

I can hardly imagine today. (And I promise to keep you informed every step of the way.) It's a commitment to constantly keeping an open mind and building and rebuilding skills in an ever-evolving environment.

KNEES TO THE LEFT . . . KNEES TO THE RIGHT . . . KNEES ALL AROUND . . .

About 99 percent of what I do now is knees. I'll occasionally let friends or former patients sneak in with other ailments, but I focus on the knee and arthroscopic procedures for it, which is my specialty. I don't do the joint replacements that I did early on in my career; I "operate" more in the arthroscopic/sports medicine world. If somebody's knees are completely shot and everything else fails, then a knee replacement is warranted and I'll recommend one of my partners or somebody who's really good for just the joint replacement. But my goal always is to try to keep people on their own knees as long as possible, and we are going to share lots of great new technology in these pages that helps me to do just that, along with the biomechanical and lifestyle tools that are perfect for any part of your frame.

KNEEPAD

A movie about my youth might be called *Sprains, Strains, and Automobiles.*

I'm into cartilage regeneration big-time right now, and sure wish it had been around when I blew out my left knee playing tackle football on the beach in my late teens. You might recall that was the same time and place for my back woes, the topic of the previous edition in this series. It's no secret that I played hard at multiple sports when I was an invincible young man, and that I still push myself when it comes to exercise and recreation. I have my share of injuries because I was a serious athlete in my

JOINT DISCUSSION

The first significant injury that really laid me up was the one I got playing football on a beach during my college years. It wasn't just touch (considering my inborn intent and that of the crowd I ran with, it could never be); it was what we called rough touch that was indistinguishable at times from full-on tackle. I was in my usual position as quarterback, and the injury was a fluke: I dropped back to throw a pass, and somebody came from the side and clipped me by accident. My knee buckled inward, and he rolled on top of me as I fell to the ground. Although it was many, many years ago, the memory is still quite vivid. (Extreme pain has a way of embedding itself well into our memory banks.)

The knee was swollen and sore as all get-out, so off to the orthopedist's office I went. Back then, they stuck everything in a cast, and I'll never forget the one I got. I lost an entire summer to that knee injury and couldn't go to the beach because it was just too hot and you don't want to get sweat and sand in the cast—it itched plenty enough all on its own. We now know (as I've said before and shall say until the cows come home) that joints, including the knee—especially the knee—need to move for nourishment. If you immobilize it too long, there are negative effects on the articular cartilage, which is the joint's cushion and shock absorber during movement.

I was in a cast longer than necessary by today's standards. I remember how loose the cast got, and that they even had to change it once because it was flopping around so much the tape they tried for a while couldn't hold it in place any longer. Looking back on what happened to me, I can tell, based upon my clinical experience looking at x-rays and other scans (the body often leaves telltale clues), that I probably had a fracture dislocation of my patella (kneecap) and a partially torn medial collateral ligament (MCL). This initial trauma long ago set me up for lots of issues down the line, and that's one of the big risk factors for knee problems (a topic included in Step 1). As for me and that new companion affixed to my leg, it felt like an eternity had passed before they buzz-sawed it off. I recovered in line with prevailing expectations of the day, but I sure didn't expect that I wouldn't recognize my leg—it was missing the majority of its usual muscle! It looked like I had polio.

Yes, certain things had healed, but I couldn't lift my own leg off the table, and I woefully limped out of the doctor's office, barely hearing the "you'll be fine" offered by the surgeon.

The doctors hadn't had me doing any exercise while I was "casted," and they didn't put me on an exercise program afterwards, either. There was no rehab program, and I was on my own like everyone else who had experienced a similar injury. I was active and athletic as much as possible (I went through a lot of trial and error about what I could and couldn't tolerate), and my knee came back after a few months.

I went on to play a pretty high level of tennis as well as martial arts—black belt and all. I did great through my twenties and into my early thirties, and then, while playing tennis one day, I started to get a little swelling in the knee. If I really overloaded it from then on, it would go sour on me and I'd have to nurse it back slowly. When I was in the latter part of my thirties, I would have to take a day off after 2 days of skiing because I would be sore, and my knee would be tight. I was grateful that I was still able to do what I wanted to do most of the time.

I went on taking time off here, or cutting back there. The "here" and "there" was much more frequent by the time I reached my midforties; I found myself altering my activities and saying no to certain things on a constant basis. Now, in my fifties, there's a serious arthritic area behind the kneecap. The main part of the joint is okay, but the kneecap feels like there's broken glass or Rice Krispies in there when I move it.

youth and am still a serious competitor well into my fifth decade. I played lots of sports as a kid, so I always got banged up, shattered my collarbone once, and had too many deep bruises, sprains, strains, and "pops" to count. But I can still play high-level tennis because I do the work on my frame that is necessary to keep me in the game.

For me, it's always about *motion* as well as medicine.

ARTICULAR CARTILAGE PARTICULARS

One of the most interesting things about articular cartilage (the joint surface cushion) is that it has a memory. When you traumatize a joint, it might look fine the day after the injury. Heck, if somebody had stuck a scope in my knee after that day at the beach that was no day at the beach, the joint cushion might have looked fine. Five years later it still might have looked fine. But research has proven that chondrocyte cells (what cartilage consists of) have a memory and can go downhill and deteriorate prematurely without any warning. That memory can come back to haunt you. I hit that point where the cells probably started dying as a result of the original impact, which was followed by a lot of overload that I am prone to apply. (Old habits

sure are hard to break. I'm one of the people who went through the no-pain, no-gain period and pushed my body really hard.)

In addition to passing on a wealth of useful knowledge about orthopedic medicine that I've acquired over more than 3 decades, I like to think that I provide an example for a lot of things relative to biomechanics generally and knees specifically. My knee was compromised because we didn't know back then that long periods of immobilization were not only unnecessary but also potentially harmful to the long-term health of the joint; I also didn't need to get so weak before coming back. Not rehabbing after injury as well as the delayed response that we sometimes see regarding articular cartilage caught up with me, and now I really have to change what I do on a daily basis. I'm still active—I play tennis every chance I get—but I pay for it sometimes, too. Trust me: I need to use just about every approach set forth in the FrameWork Knee Program.

I practice medicine and I do the things I like to do in my free time, and I am realistic

KNEEPAD

Articular cartilage has limited self-repair ability—for now.

about what can and can't be fixed at this point. I have a lot of patients with knee conditions similar to mine, and some keep going from doctor to doctor and then around the horn back to me because they're looking for answers that aren't available yet. I've lost the cushion in my joint, and although we can regenerate portions of the cushion in certain instances now, the technology is just not quite there to repave the road, which is what I need under my knee. We can fill potholes if you have focal areas of loss or degeneration; if we look into a knee and see a pothole brewing, we can now sometimes regenerate the cushion and rebalance the kneecap using a variety of techniques. That might have been really helpful to me when I was in my thirties and symptoms appeared, and maybe I wouldn't be where I am right now, but facts are facts—I'm beyond help for certain procedures.

But not beyond the help provided by a comprehensive program that is designed to make the most of what I have and avoid, or at least put off indefinitely, more drastic surgical measures.

As for my other knee, the right one, I think I must have been set up for problems with it because you don't usually dislocate a kneecap like I did unless there's some predisposing tilt on the kneecap or instability or looseness of the kneecap. If you have tilt or laxity, you can develop issues even without blunt trauma. My opposite knee has developed some similar symptoms that, thankfully, are not as bad as they are in the left one. On "balance," it seems to me that I was an accident waiting to happen. Again, prevention could have made all the difference.

Articular cartilage was one of my early areas of interest, and it still is today. My initial surgical training included a year spent doing basic science research, and I was one of the early researchers who worked on storing articular cartilage and transplanting it, trying to regenerate joint cushions. We would take a piece of joint off, try to regrow it, and then put it back in to see what happened. That's exactly what has come to fruition now; we're starting to see this science and technology at a point where it's paying off in many knee cases. While it's too late for me, I use it often when confronted by knee cushion problems that are legion (see Step 2).

KNEEPAD

We can fill potholes if you have focal areas of cartilage degeneration. We can't yet repave the road.

JOINT DISCUSSION

Orthopedic researchers who worked with knees many years ago discovered that articular cartilage (the joint cushion) is very unique tissue and had little, if any, repair capability. One researcher said that if you opened up a knee and carved your initials in the shiny smooth cushion, and then took a look inside 20 years later, you would still see your marks there as you would when initials are carved in tree bark.

Medical terminology can be confusing, and the knee is no exception. In addition to the articular cartilage, there is another type of cartilage, the meniscus (there will be a lot more about cartilage and other knee anatomy in Step 1). Like articular cartilage, it has a very limited blood supply and very limited healing capability. For a long time we thought there wasn't much we could do for a damaged or torn meniscus; we now know that there are some promising repairs that can be effected that are short of removal. (Because the meniscus is one of the main protectors of the knee, saving it can be the difference between a healthy, functioning knee 10 or 20 years later, and a beat-up arthritic knee.) We also know we can learn a lot more about how to enhance whatever capability the meniscus has for repair. Scientists are trying a few things that we'll cover in Step 2, and we include some experimental but very promising approaches in the Afterword that frame the future of knee treatment.

Fear not—we're saving more of Mother Nature's original equipment every day. We try to catch defects earlier and, if appropriate, resurface them a little or fill the pothole and allow some cushion to grow back slowly over time. When possible, we actually repair the meniscus rather than remove it. These types of interventions will prevent arthritis from occurring, and that's pretty amazing in itself. There's a lot of research going into this right now, and I expect breakthroughs will be steady in the near future.

UNFAIR TO THE FAIRER SEX

There's been an exponential increase of knee injuries in females, and we'll go into that in great depth in Step 1. Suffice to say, women are at uncommon risk for a variety of reasons, and they experience five to seven times the rate of certain serious knee injuries that their male counterparts do. These young women are going to join the arthritic brigades in their thirties, forties, and fifties.

Preconditions, or setups as I refer to them, are one of the big concerns I have with young female athletes. I'm all for women being fit and achieving and playing high-level sports (need I mention again the many benefits of vigorous exercise?); the big "but" here is, is it a smart thing for droves of young women to be in sports that pose high risks to the knees, such as soccer, field hockey, lacrosse, and basketball, if their knee injury rates are off the chart? I don't have the answer, but I also don't think this question is being explored and tossed around enough.

My whole life I've been into fitness and talked about fitness equality for everybody, as well as getting kids active and fit, but there's a difference between being active and fit and going out and exposing yourself to a high-risk sport if your body's not ready for it. That's the big "if" that goes with the big "but." It's not enough to get back to where you were before an injury; you have to be better than 100 percent. You have to have new abilities with that knee and its support structure, or you're probably going to reinjure it.

FRAMEWORK REFRAMED

A couple of years ago I published a comprehensive program that addressed all of the body's muscles, bones, and joints—everything you need to live life to the fullest. One of its keys for developing and keeping a healthy frame was building core strength. However, your core is not just six-pack abs; it's your back muscles, oblique muscles, hips, pelvis, and thighs, and if we connect those dots, guess where you end up?

The knees.

You can't walk, climb, run, change direction, or sit without them, and you're going to do one or more of those every day whether your knees hurt or they don't (unless, of course, you plan to stay immobile indefinitely). It behooves us to do everything we can to build them up and shore them up, and that process doesn't only involve the knees themselves. You must address things from the ground up—all the way to the executive suite otherwise known as your brain.

The fact is, sedentary is not an option for anyone (yes, I said that before, too). Being idle is as dangerous for your health as smoking a pack of cigarettes a day. Being active over the long haul requires a frame that is flexible, strong, durable, and balanced. It's all well and good to have "mirror muscles" or advanced running capability, but if your entire frame isn't in shape, you're a candidate for aches and pulls and sprains, for joint dysfunctions and arthritis, and for diminished mobility.

Being active and achieving optimal health also means being pain free, or at least in pain "health"—able to live with it and move around in spite of it. Your eyes will open wide when you discover how different, and better, your life is after you pay a little attention to your hinges.

The knee program, though specialized as the back program is, is designed to work within the context of overall *biomechanical* health. It makes little sense to get your knee back into shape, or work to keep it in shape or improve its performance, if the rest of your frame that is connected to it is out of shape or out of whack. How individual parts are connected determines how well you function, and how you experience pain. Take the six steps outlined in subsequent chapters if you want to maximize the former and minimize the latter.

If you have made a commitment to core fitness (outlined in the original *FrameWork*), then you are ready to reap the benefits of the *FrameWork for the Knee* program. In Step 1,

Knee Deep, we'll familiarize you with the basic anatomy of the knee, the bones and cushions and bands, and how they were designed to deliver proprioception (fine-tune coordination, for those of you who didn't pay close enough attention earlier). Included in this step is a survey of the weak links that have the potential to cause problems. All of the things that can go wrong with those anatomical parts, and how they can best be fixed, are covered in the next step, Woe Is Knee.

Following the template established in the last book, Step 3: "Knoodle" This is a fun self-check of your overall health and fitness, especially in relation to your knees, and an assessment of just what kind of shape your knees are really in. "Kneed" to Know—all of the lifestyle issues that impact health no matter which part of the frame we're discussing—is Step 4.

The next step is the pièce de résistance: the knee workouts that fit any circumstance—Beginner/Recovery, Intermediate, or Advanced—with special exercise modifications and suggestions for the most common knee ailments. It's been said (and I wish that were by me), "If all of the benefits of exercise could be packaged in a single pill, it would be the most prescribed medication in the world." Whatever shape your knees are in, they'll be a whole lot better after a focused routine.

We wrap things up with a few prescriptive directions for the most troublesome knees in Step 6: "Kneed" More? and then look toward the future in the Afterword.

Changes in your body are inevitable; problems aren't. Everything you need is here for the taking so that you can live the way you're supposed to.

ACTIVE FOR LIFE

Any machine, including the human one, will lose efficiency and break down at some point. Of all the people who have lived past the age of 65, two-thirds are alive today, so it's no shock that musculoskeletal ailments leapfrogged the common cold around the year 2000 as the number-one reason for doctor visits. Problems with muscles, bones, and joints fill many physicians' schedules, driven in no small measure by knee problems in all of their forms. This is where biomechanics— how body parts work in conjunction with each other—comes in.

I'll say it again: I'm all about *motion* and the medicine that pertains to it. I'll repeat as well that whatever shape you're in now, it can be better. You can move about better, you can

recreate better, you can have a better foundation for later years. How?

With an intention to do it and a commitment to regular exercise, because motion is about mind-set, too.

You have desires and expectations for the best of health, but you've also got responsibilities in securing and maintaining it. Being lean and beautiful on the outside isn't enough. You've got to have a structure that's going to support you tomorrow and the next day and the day after. The immutable truth is, people who do more live longer.

The arthroscope led me to the knee and then to sports medicine, where it first gained promi-

KNEEPAD

"Active for Life" Goals

Flexibility	Balance
Strength	Durability

nence. Playing sports at a high competitive level was an early love, and sports are still a personal passion that dovetails with my professional one. Sports are the epitome of *action,* and I'm passionate about helping you to stay active—on any level, from walking around the block to skiing cross-country, even snowboarding—for life.

Knee Deep

Before embarking on any biomechanical training program, having a basic understanding of the parts involved is more than useful—it's critical. You have to know what's involved with movement so you can understand *why* you should be faithful to the exercises that keep your components humming. And when you know why, your brain will be fully engaged to balance the mind/body component of good health. Yes, the practice of mind-fulness can be applied to keeping your knees healthy and functioning optimally.

I know I'm partial, but the knee is truly amazing. When I look at sports players who put up with so much every day, and yet don't get injured, I marvel at how ingenious its design is. They, and their knees, jump, twist, pivot, change direction, and land, often seemingly off-balance, at warp speed. One needs to watch the slow motion replays to fully appreciate what has occurred; in fact, there are computerized high-speed biomechanical analysis tools that we now use to better understand the complex biomechanical movement patterns unique to each sport. When all of the parts are fine-tuned, amazing athletic feats are possible for some and the rest of us can get around reasonably well without toppling over.

So without further ado, and mindful of keeping the academics to a minimum, let's "scope" the knee together.

View of Knee from Front

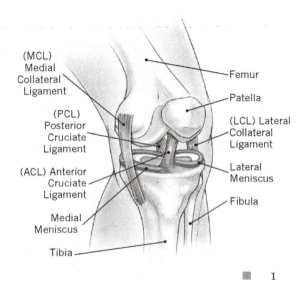

THE BARE BONES

When people think about the knee, they usually just think about the kneecap, or patella, or a simple hinge structure. However, it takes more than one part to make a hinge, and the knee is even more complex than that. It consists of two distinct joints formed by three bones: the patella and femur (thigh bone) get up close and personal in the patellofemoral joint; and the femur and the tibia (leg bone) do likewise in the tibiofemoral one.

The main part of your knee is where the femur and tibia meet; it's the main hinge that is loaded most of the time when you stand, walk, or run, especially on level surfaces. This tibiofemoral area is made up of two compartments: the inner (medial) and the outer (lateral). The patellofemoral area provides the third compartment of the knee, and this is formed by the kneecap and thigh bone. The area of the thighbone that houses the kneecap is called the trochlea. The patellofemoral joint is loaded and relied on even more when the knee is flexed, like when you go up and down stairs, ski, or do squats and lunges at the gym. The patella is interesting in that it is a bone that lives within a muscle-tendon complex, something we call a sesamoid bone (you have a few others of these around your frame). This

is a smart design from a biomechanical standpoint in that it increases tendon leverage on the femur during leg extension. It is also a setup for a variety of unique problems that can occur around the oft-temperamental kneecap.

When healthy, these three compartments work in unison, smoothly gliding across each other with a coefficient of friction *20 times* more slippery than ice on ice. But there are some thorny design problems that are unique to the knee, and when things go wrong, the grinding starts. It can be throughout the entire knee, involving all three compartments equally, or the problem can be selective and isolated to just one or two of the compartments. I'm a perfect example. My main tibiofemoral area is pretty good, but, from my old injury, my patellofemoral articulation is shot, pretty much bone on bone, awaiting the parts department.

In addition to the bony architecture, there are plenty of other "softer" things that can run afoul in the knee.

THE SOFTER SIDE

Ligaments, tendons, and muscles all play a role in knee design, but cartilage tops the list when it comes to picking a lead actor. What will surprise many of you is that there are two kinds: articular cartilage (it looks like the smooth white opaque ball that you might recall seeing at the end of a chicken bone), and the meniscus (fibrocartilage) that most lay people have in mind when they refer to a torn knee cartilage. They are two completely different components. Perhaps this is imprecise terminology, but it's important to appreciate the distinction.

Side View of Knee from Outer (Lateral) Side

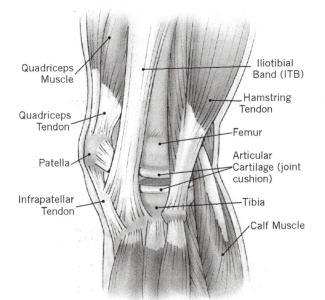

Quadriceps Muscle

Quadriceps Tendon

Patella

Infrapatellar Tendon

Iliotibial Band (ITB)

Hamstring Tendon

Femur

Articular Cartilage (joint cushion)

Tibia

Calf Muscle

■ ARTICULAR CARTILAGE

This frame part is a smooth joint surface cushion that covers the ends of both the tibiofemoral and the patellofemoral joints (or any joint in your body for that matter). It's sort of a cap on the end of the bone surfaces that functions as a cushion so that bone-on-bone doesn't occur. When healthy, the articular cartilage is thick and smooth and looks like newly polished white marble. When damaged, it can start to look like a shag carpet, and if it wears all the way down, you can actually see the bone, or even have a bone-on-bone situation. You will hear more about arthritis (which is a wearing down of the articular cartilage) as well as chondral defects, which are focal areas of damage (like "potholes") in the articular cartilage cushion. When your cushion is damaged, it is often the beginning of the end for your knee. (Unless, of course, you do something about it.)

■ MENISCI

The meniscus is a shock absorber and space filler that consists of rubbery material akin to the body of a clam. It's C-shaped, and there's one on both the

KNEEPAD

medial (inner) and lateral (outer) sides of the knee. The two menisci are appropriately called the medial meniscus and lateral meniscus.

Menisci are protectors of knee joints, and they're critical for knee congruity and stability because they help create a perfect fit for the articular cartilage cushions of the femur and tibia as they glide and twist across each other. For that reason, we now do everything we can to preserve and protect the meniscus after a knee injury, or during knee surgery, rather than a few years back where, as I said before, the goal was usually to remove the whole thing. One more critical point: Because the menisci are slick and pliable to minimize friction, they're critical for pain-free motion.

LIGAMENTS

Your knee and its shock absorbers are kept in place by four primary knee ligaments, or taut bands. There's one on the inner side of the knee (the medial collateral ligament, or MCL) and one on the outer side (the lateral collateral ligament, or LCL) that prevent side-to-side drift. To keep abnormal front-back movement in check, the posterior cruciate ligament (PCL) and the (infamous) anterior cruciate ligament (ACL) crisscross (hence the name "cruciate") in the center of the knee.

The four major knee ligaments work in concert to prevent abnormal movement patterns within the knee. Interestingly, almost like strings on a tennis racquet, we are all "strung" with a little different tension; some of us have very tight ligaments, and others (especially females) are more "loose-jointed." If your ligaments are loose, you might do better in yoga class or in the circus, but you are at higher risk for a variety of injuries.

TENDONS

Several additional taut bands support front-back stability as they expand and contract with motion: The quadriceps tendon attaches the quadriceps or thigh muscle to the upper part of the patella; the infrapatellar tendon connects the lower part of the patella to the tibia (at an area called the tibial tubercle); and the hamstring tendons run across the back of the knee on both the medial and lateral side. (The calf muscle runs up the lower leg and actually also attaches up behind the knee.)

ILIOTIBIAL BAND (ITB)

The ITB consists of fibrous tissue that is similar to a tendon. It's wide and long, traveling from the upper leg muscles of the outer thigh area, across the lateral side of the knee, to the tibia below, where it attaches.

MUSCLES

The leg muscles are the pistons and driveshaft, if you will, of the knee machine.

KNEEPAD

Combined, the quadriceps and its tendon, and the patellar and the infrapatellar tendons are called the extensor mechanism of the knee and function as the major muscle-tendon group for it. It's a common source of knee problems for adolescents and young athletes.

You can be sure the quadriceps, hamstring, and calf muscles that are a part of every FrameWork program will be given particular attention in this one because of their connections to knee health.

And it doesn't stop there. We are learning that even core and pelvic musculature are critical in maintaining optimal knee function and preventing knee injuries.

NEUROMUSCULAR CONTROL

Last (but hardly least when it comes to frame work) is what links all of the above individual anatomical parts together to perform like an orchestra, rather than a group of soloists: neuromuscular factors, a combination of nerves and muscle activity that interacts with the spinal cord and brain, giving your knee and you agility—that proprioception (fine-tune coordination) that we have stressed and will continue to explore in this book. Optimal neuromuscular function is something that can be trained (and lost with injury, casting, aging, or inactivity), and is every bit as important as any major ligament or muscle when it comes to keeping knees healthy for life.

"JUST A LITTLE DAB WILL DO YA"

There's a final ingredient in the inner workings of Mother Nature's hinge: magical fluid. An undetectable drop of this synovial fluid (the lining of the knee is called the synovium)—which is all you should have in your knee—just one drop of this awesome WD-40-like lubricant glistens all joint surfaces and carries far more than its weight when it comes to that better-than-ice coefficient mentioned previously. (Anyone who recognizes the title of this section is old enough to be concerned about this fluid because "drying up" is an issue in collagen and brain cells, along with some other cells, as we age.) Synovial fluid also has some components that help nourish and protect the articular cartilage joint cushion, which has no intrinsic blood supply, so it relies on the synovial fluid for its nourishment. Movement and exercise enhance this process by pumping synovial fluid into the cushion. Hence my mantra, "motion is lotion." In knees with arthritis, the synovial fluid becomes less viscous and is not as good a lubricant as it is supposed to be.

WEAK LINKS

When evaluating a knee case, I always take into account the patient's predisposition toward whatever ailment that presents. Weak links are one of the common threads in this series because they play a role in every aspect of frame health, and they are always part of the frank discussion I have about a knee issue. Time is not a factor when I explain that many of the things that interfere with knee health and function, causing one complaint or another, can be corrected by the patient him- or herself, and that those that are beyond his or her control can usually be managed.

JOINT DISCUSSION

I have knee patients work on the calf, along with the hamstrings, quadriceps, and hip abductors and adductors. The calf is an assist muscle, especially going up and down stairs. When people have a bad knee like mine, it's so worn that steps and stairs hurt. My body compensates and my calves wind up bigger than they should be (balance, remember?), so instead of using my quad to spring upwards, I use the foot press more than I should. (Sometimes, in response to pain or other brain signals, your amazing body will make little adjustments that might not result in the best biomechanics.)

AGE

This is listed first because every age presents its own set of knee problems: Growing children have one part or another that is loose as they mature, and it's not uncommon that a growth plate in a knee bone is waiting around for soft tissue to catch up; mature people have initial wear and tear (with or without symptoms) that will spread unless serious intervention ensues; seniors are candidates for more advanced arthritis and certain fractures with their concomitant issues.

In addition to the above specifics, there are some general consequences of aging that threaten every frame:

- Probability of injury increases

- Severity of injury increases

- Time to heal increases

- Degree of healing decreases

- Cellular and biochemical changes occur:
  - Bone loses density
  - Ligaments weaken
  - Growth hormone production decreases
  - Collagen is lost and its structural integrity diminished
  - Neural loss (neuromuscular wiring goes from cable high-speed to dial-up)
  - Muscle mass and strength diminish, as does reaction time
  - Loss of proprioception

All this adds up to higher vulnerability. Yessiree—age is a biggie when it comes to knees, and it's so big, the next section is devoted entirely to what can go wrong with our knees from our youth on up to our twilight years.

GENDER

A weak link affecting half of the population explains a large percentage of the cases I see all the time, so it merits a corresponding share of a knee discussion.

It's been proven that up until puberty, boys and girls land the same way from jumps, and from then on, girls start landing differently: Their knees either buckle in slightly or they land more stiff-legged—they're not landing like a cat anymore. (They have a landing gear problem whereby the knees don't transfer as much shock as they should.)

JOINT DISCUSSION

Knee MRI studies involving the over-60 crowd showed significant issues in the majority of patients, even those without symptoms. Scans of the interior of their menisci showed that, instead of appearing black as healthy menisci do, there was a whitish-grayish material in the center that indicated fatty degeneration. (This was similar to findings on the spinal intervertebral disks we talked about in the previous book about the lower back.) It doesn't take much to go from there to an actual separation of tissue, which we refer to as a degenerative tear. (It's like a tear in a pair of pants—certain movements and twists, even regular ones like a golf swing, will spread it. So a meniscus tear propagates with age and becomes more and more symptomatic.) These types of meniscal tears are very common with aging (as multiple MRI studies have shown), and like gray hair and wrinkles, not all need treatment. Each case must be individualized.

The different biomechanics and landings may be because women have a slightly wider pelvis; at puberty, girls start to mature, and the angles around the knee are a little different. There may be muscular, strength, or hormonal issues at play, too. Females are also more loose-jointed, and that's another risk factor they have for knee problems.

Once again, proprioception is critical. When a female (or anyone else, for that matter) sprains an ankle and thinks it's all better shortly thereafter, but it keeps spraining, fine-tune coordination hasn't been fully reestablished. The same is true for the knee. The FrameWork Knee Program takes care of that for anyone who hasn't had the benefit of special training, such as dancers who learn how to land properly when they jump. (At a very young age, fantastic proprioception is imbedded in the muscle and nerve memory of their knees).

The agility drills we put women through now accomplish the same thing, and we have reduced anterior cruciate ligament (ACL) tear rates by more than 50 percent for high school and college athletes who play high-risk sports. It amazes me that every single sports team in our

JOINT DISCUSSION

We know that all too often ACL tears are not just an accident. In fact, they are somewhat predictable. Both genetics and gender play a role, and I am reminded of two families that I have treated surgically for ACL reconstructions over the years. They have also become friends, and I can tell you without hesitation that they would much rather see me socially at this point in time than in my office. Both families illustrate the role that genetics play in ACL tears. One mom, a wonderful veterinarian, came to me when she tore her own ACL. The surgery went great and she had a full recovery. We saw much more of each other when her teenage daughter tore both her right and her left ACL. In between, she also managed to dislocate a kneecap. Not only do ACL tears run in families, but if you tear one, we now know that you are also at higher risk of tearing the other. The other mother (of three teenagers) came to me when her teenage son tore his ACL. One month later, her teenage daughter did the same thing. When her third son injured his knee months later, I was thrilled to inform her that it was only a minor MCL sprain and he did not need surgery. He recovered fully and returned to sports—but also went on to tear his ACL the following year! I really felt for these moms and their families. They seemed to take things in stride (I hope I was able to help that process), and I remember the mother of three smiling and saying, "Tic-tac-toe, three in a row."

KNEEPAD

There are programs now for retraining young athletes (and older ones, too) to jump and land properly, more agilely, with more proprioception around the knee—that fine-tune coordination we've emphasized. Santa Monica Orthopaedic and Sports Medicine Group (www.aclprevent .com) offers an excellent one; check your local listings because these are coming to more neighborhoods all the time.

JOINT DISCUSSION

I've been fortunate to work with dancers at all levels for 27 years, including those who performed for the Pennsylvania Ballet. There aren't many "dance doctors" like me, so we usually get patients from a large geographical area.

Dancers come to me from Europe, from all over, really, and I almost never see ACL tears in them. One would think, as I did, that dancers should be at high risk for these tears, and yet, over almost 3 decades, I can count on one hand the number of such tears I've seen. On the other hand, there were times when I've done ACLs for what seemed like an entire basketball, soccer, or field hockey team of high school girls in only one season. What was going on with those dancers? I often wondered. Why are these extremely loose-jointed, high-risk females, who are jumping and landing day in and day out, protected, as if they were immunized from the dreaded ACL tear?

After only a couple of years of treating dancers, I was puzzled enough to pick up the phone and call Bill Hamilton, the most famous dance doctor in the world, who treated Baryshnikov and members of the New York City Ballet and the American Ballet Theatre. "Bill," I said, "you've treated dancers longer than me, many more than I have seen or will ever see in my life. Let me ask you: How many ACL tears have you come across?" I could almost see him scratching his head before he replied.

"You know, Nick, I know I've had a few, but honestly, I can't recall many at all."

So I called the Pittsburgh Ballet doc, the Houston Ballet doc, and a few others. Every one said the same thing to me. I asked myself: Is it a different type and level of activity that dancers engage in from a very young age that immunizes them? After all, they start when they're 2 or 3 and they have to learn to jump and land correctly. They're trained so well that they can probably do it blindfolded or in their sleep, and they do it all the time, so they're physically powerful as well as flexible. Dancers are the epitome of core strength (where have we heard that before?), and I knew that, among its many benefits, core fitness helps protect the ACL and the kneecap.

Not long after my initial inquiries, I talked to a couple of researchers who had big labs where ACL injury research (sophisticated jumping and landing analysis) was being done. I asked them to study 12-year-old female dancers and non-dancers and tell me how each test group lands, because I more than suspected that the dancers land like males do, before and after puberty. To my dismay, nobody wanted to do this controlled experiment.

Flash forward about 2 decades to the latter part of 2009. A medical article that came out of New York City claimed that dancers are much less likely to tear an ACL. I'm thinking about giving the authors a call to ask where the impetus for that great idea came from. Might they have heard me bang that particular drum over the years? Either way, there's a lot we can learn from dancers, or as Yogi Berra said, "You can observe a lot by watching."

---

nation (especially the higher-risk female sports) has not mandated these successful preventive programs (coaches, listen up here) because they also improve sports performance!

Proprioception can be trained, or retrained as the case may be, and it must be if you want to keep your frame healthy and your life active. Otherwise, everyone is at risk for tears and re-tears in one knee, and tears in the other knee because of biomechanical compensation and other intrinsic predisposing factors—something we see too often for my liking. It's not enough to get back to where you were before the injury; you have to have the most proprioception you can get (stick around for Step 5). You really have to be "bet-ter than 100 percent" in terms of recovery after an ACL injury or surgery, something that most patients (and often their parents and coaches) have a hard time grasping.

SUBPAR OVERALL FITNESS

Again, no frame part operates independently in your body, so it stands to reason that if you're out of shape generally, you'll have specific ailments sooner or later. We've covered this until the cows came home; nonetheless, there are certain things that just can't be considered too much (like the information in Step 4: "Kneed" to Know):

Sedentary Lifestyle

Many of us spend huge chunks of our day at a desk or on our feet without moving about much, and lower backs aren't the only frame part that can stiffen as a result. Knees can, and do, tighten up to the point where sudden, albeit normal, movement can cause something to overextend or even snap.

Aerobic Condition

Muscles need oxygen like engines need gas; they and other soft tissue need a vigorous blood supply to stay healthy. If they get less-than-ideal nourishment, they weaken and the support they were designed to provide is compromised. The result is increased vulnerability to breakdown.

Imbalances

Fitness fanatics who run or work out religiously in the gym, or who hit the courts and playing fields every week, are prone to having an overworked frame part that taxes other ones abnormally. Imbalances can develop in their frames as a direct result of

KNEEPAD

Weak Links

Aging EFX	Overweight
Gender	Old injuries
Subpar overall fitness	Incomplete rehab
Frame imbalances	Genetics

their activity or sport, something I see all the time. These imbalances could also result when rehabbing or compensating for an injured part, as in my own case. Optimal biomechanics relies on form, function, and force; imbalance in any part of the motion equation could break the chain of health at any time.

OVERWEIGHT

This imbalance merits separate treatment because of its prevalence today. The more your frame has to support, the harder it has to work and the more susceptible it is to injury. (There's plenty on this subject for you to chew on later.)

OLD INJURIES

Your body is just like paper, metal, and wood: Its cracks and tears and breaks can be "glued," "taped," "stapled," or "welded," but it may never be as strong as it was originally. If you want to avoid a "Groundhog Day" injury experience, pay special attention to the elements that impact your future mobility:

- Incomplete rehabilitation

- Strenuous recreation too soon

- Improper warmup of affected area

- Poor nutritional support

- Overtraining and/or overuse syndromes

- Medication camouflage of symptoms

All of the above can be detrimental to your recovery and increase susceptibility to re-injury.

GENETICS

Everyone is born with a pedigree that leads to structural anomalies or systemic deficiencies. (I suppose genetics are the ultimate predisposition we all have.) If you're bowlegged or knock-kneed, you're

going to wear down the medial or lateral compartment of the knee, respectively; if connective tissue is shorter or longer than normal, you're more vulnerable to sprains, tears, and snaps. Some people have genetic indicators for arthritis, heart disease, obesity, or pain, and there are plenty who haven't been given a fair complement of athletic prowess. When it comes to knees, all of this must be taken into account. (This is where "management" comes to the fore.) The best advice I can give is to choose your parents wisely, and short of that, remember that your genetics may be the hand you are dealt, but as any good poker player will tell you, it's also about how you play the cards. I am one who believes that it is never too late to change your fate.

GROWING PAINS

Thankfully, the overwhelming majority of knee aches are not surgical emergencies, but they usually are (or will be) serious enough to demand attention and a proper evaluation. While some conditions—patellar pain, overuse injury, stress fracture—can happen to anyone at any age, some complaints are associated more with one age group than with the others. (Except for a couple of exceptions below, treatments are covered in the next chapter.)

One important point to start with is that there really is no such thing as growing pains. It does not hurt to grow, but growth, especially when it is rapid, can create certain muscle imbalances and other issues that might predispose the growing frame to painful problems. Some of the following conditions are the usual suspects when growing frames start to moan.

The Childhood Frame

I see kids of all ages who have knee problems, and most of them are caused by overuse of a joint and support structure that is still developing:

Patellar Pain Syndrome

Also sometimes known as runner's knee or chondromalacia, this is a result of the kneecap rubbing against one side of the joint, which irritates and overloads the articular cartilage underneath. Pain occurs when walking up or down stairs, kneeling, squatting, or sitting with a bent knee for a long period of time.

A number of factors can contribute to patellar pain:

- Malalignment of the kneecap and/or leg

- Patellar tendon dislocation or subluxation (partial dislocation)

- Patellar tendon hypermobility (loose-jointed)

- Injury

- Excessive training or overuse

- Tightness, imbalance, or weakness of thigh, core, and pelvic muscles

- Inadequate stretching

- Flat feet

Patellar pain is not a serious knee problem, but it can be a very disabling one, and one that is a real challenge for the patient, the patient's family, and the treating physician. I liken it to the "migraine headache" of the knee. As with migraines, x-rays and MRIs are often normal, but the pain can be severe. Also like people with migraines, patients with patellar pain need to try to identify the activity-related triggers that set off symptoms. Surgery does not have the best results for patellar pain, and in most cases it should be considered as a last resort. There are many excellent preventive programs, with exercise and exercise modification the mainstay approaches. As a knee specialist, I probably have more gray hairs from managing patients with this condition than any other, but I am also very understanding and sympathetic, as I personally have this same condition, a more advanced degenerative state related to my old knee trauma. (More on the wayward patella in later sections, as there is much overlap in the child and adult versions of this complaint.)

Osgood-Schlatter Disease (OSD)

Osgood-Schlatter Disease is not really a "disease" but rather a condition characterized by tenderness, swelling, and soreness of the tibial tuberosity (the upper part of the tibia just below the kneecap, where the patellar tendon attaches). A firm, painful bump actually can appear a few inches below the kneecap in the uppermost part of the shinbone. OSD presents mostly in children between the ages of 9 and 16 who play sports on a regular basis and are undergoing a growth spurt. The tuberosity, or apophysis, gets overloaded and splits a tad,

similar to a stress (or "hairline") fracture. It tries to heal itself and gets a little thicker, and that new growth solidifies and often stays there. Usually, the pain goes away when adult height is achieved; rarely, pain persists even after one is fully grown. There are many simple treatments and preventive programs that keep kids with OSD active, although they will sometimes need to be slowed down when symptoms get more severe.

Epiphyseal Fracture

A growth plate (also known as an epiphysis) on the end of long bones like the femur and tibia near the knee is especially vulnerable to a complete or partial break, or abnormal compres-

KNEEPAD

Childhood Knee Conditions

Patellar Pain Syndrome (Chondromalacia Patella)

Osgood-Schlatter Disease

Epiphyseal (Growth Plate) Fracture

Osteochondritis Dissecans

Ligament Tear

Discoid Lateral Meniscus

Juvenile Rheumatoid Arthritis (JRA)

sion, because the surrounding ligaments are stronger than newly forming bone at the growth plate. A chain will always break at its weakest link, and in growing children, the growth plates are often weaker than the collateral ligaments, so the epiphysis takes the brunt of the trauma and that's what gives way.

Osteochondritis Dissecans (OCD)

This condition affects teenagers and young adults, especially those active in sports, and we still do not know its exact cause. It may be secondary to trauma, or, similar to Perthes Disease of the hip, it may be caused by a vascular problem whereby the blood supply to a localized area within the knee joint is cut off. The affected area of bone, including an area of the joint cushion or articular cartilage, might stay in place, or a fragment might break away and cause significant problems. Some heal spontaneously; others require major surgery to restore the joint cushion or even regenerate it, so that arthritis, at a young age, can be prevented.

Ligament Tear

Even though we are seeing more and more of these in younger and younger kids, ligament tears are not extremely common in youngsters (meaning, before the growth spurts start), although I did see a complete ACL tear in a 9-year-old a few years back. In younger, growing kids, if it happens, it's usually the result of a traumatic injury, and sometimes it's a case where the ligament, rather than splitting into two pieces, pulls off a small piece of bone instead. Sometimes a cast will suffice, and other times the ligament or bone fragment must be surgically re-attached. After youngsters hit the teen years, there is a rapid increase in ligament tears like the dreaded ACL one, especially in females. (This condition and the one that follows are covered in greater depth in the next age group.)

Meniscus Tear

This ailment occurs as the consequence of an injury or as the result of degeneration related to injury or age, and sometimes it's a combination of those two factors—so it's not common that we see a meniscus tear in younger, growing kids, except for the teenagers who find ways to tear them up. A healthy person who gets whacked on the knee or twists it violently while playing sports, or a person who does repetitive squats over time, such as a baseball catcher, gardener, plumber, or auto mechanic, could experience a torn meniscus. Also, anyone who tears an ACL will often also tear a meniscus.

As we discussed earlier, a damaged meniscus will develop an internal whitish-gray area, which is a sign of weakness. (I tell patients it's like an apple that looks great on the outside, but you cut it in half and there's a big brown spot inside.) It provides less stability and shock absorption, which leads to the development of arthritis in the knee. As the arthritis progresses, the meniscus is weakened further, and it doesn't take much for the internal weakness to spread to the surface and cause a tear (these are called degenerative meniscal tears). And then, like a small rip in the seat of your pants, any wrong move will just about guarantee that the meniscus tear will get a lot worse.

This injury is also relatively rare in children, but some have a discoid lateral meniscus that was incompletely formed during embryonic development—it's round, flat, and disk-shaped, instead of C-shaped and spongy, which makes it more susceptible to injury. However, most people who have one of these, even some high-performing athletes, never know it. The ones who do report pain on the outer side of the knee, and refer to a "popping" or catching sensation on the outer side of the knee. (This is not to be confused with patellar pain syndrome and/or ITB issues, both of which also hurt on the outer or lateral side of the knee.)

Juvenile Rheumatoid Arthritis (JRA)

Kids can get arthritis or have medical issues that result in knee and other joint aches and pains. The most common type of arthritis in children under 16 years old, JRA is an autoimmune-type disorder, possibly triggered by a virus or bacteria, and it is characterized by joint stiffness, pain, and limited range of motion; the joint might also be red and warm to the touch. JRA is sometimes accompanied by a rash, fever, or swollen lymph glands, and some cases include red eyes, eye pain, and vision changes. I mention this relatively rare condition to point out that a painful, swollen knee (or knees) in children is not always a result of injury, overuse, or sport. (Lyme disease, with involvement of the knee, known as Lyme arthritis, is another example of a systemic illness—caused by a tick bite—that can present with knee pain and swelling at any age, and I've seen it quite often in kids.) A thorough doctor will consider all possibilities.

The Young Adult Frame

Next up are the almost-adults in their late teens and twenties who have pretty much reached their final height. They're vulnerable to knee woes because of the imbalances that develop naturally during growth spurts and because they play a lot harder. The mileage begins to build up, but fortunately the repair shop is in excellent working order, often functioning overtime. Young adults are proud of newfound height and strength, and they push themselves to the limit in sports and recreation. Combine that mind-set with the aforementioned imbalances that have yet to resolve themselves and—voilà!—they suffer traumatic injuries more often. (The good news—especially for guys who have lots of testosterone at this time of their lives—is that the young adult body still retains a great deal of self-healing ability. The First Aid section later on helps that along.)

Patellar Pain

It may come as a surprise to you that most of your height results from two growth plates around your knee. Those plates can take off very quickly during the final stage of your body's development and grow faster than the surrounding muscles and tendons can accommodate. So you go from being a Gumby as a kid to having a very tight hamstring and outer thigh all of a sudden, and those are set-ups for patellar pain. Unlike the achy kneecaps of younger kids, young adult patellas can sometimes already show signs of softening, wear, and/or damage if viewed with a scope or with a high-definition MRI. Otherwise, the nagging kneecap in this group is very similar in terms of the predisposing factors and treatments discussed in the following pages for younger kids and adults.

Patellar Dislocation

The patellofemoral joint is a relatively shallow joint (and some people's are more so than others), and the kneecap is prone to shifting in directions that it shouldn't. Dislocations can be the result of contact on the field of play or the result of planting a foot and twisting the knee without any contact being involved. It usually occurs laterally and is very painful. (A partial dislocation is called a subluxation.)

Susceptibility to patellar dislocation is increased by wider than normal hips (one reason it is more common in females), or a shallower than normal trochlea (that groove at the lower end of the femur). For some, the trochlea groove is so shallow that the kneecap is like an ice cube on a small plate, slipping and sliding.

Patellar Tendinitis ("Jumper's Knee")

This is another overuse injury that results from repetitive overloading of the extensor mechanism, which is the combination of muscles and tendons we discussed previously. Patellar tendinitis is a relatively common condition that begins as inflammation of the patellar tendon where it attaches to the patella and that causes pain in the anterior (front) part of the knee, at the bottom or tip of the kneecap. The pain starts as a dull ache and gradually increases over time as microtears in the tendon spread. Initially, soreness is felt after a game or workout, but as the condition worsens, pain can be constant. A tight quadriceps muscle is often one of the culprits, so early treatment involves a lot of stretching and usually some physical therapy targeting it. In addition to manipulation, therapists might also teach advanced stretching techniques using proprioceptive neuromuscular facilitation (PNF), in which contract-relax techniques are used to trick the muscle into a better stretch. Therapists might also use modalities such as ultrasound, H-Wave, or InterX stimulation.

Eccentric loading (contraction of the muscle while it is lengthening) occurs when landing from a jump or decelerating. Jumper's knee occurs in many types of athletes but is most common in sports that require explosive jumping movements, such as basketball, volleyball, ballet, and soccer. Knee loads of up to seven times one's body weight occur during a soccer kick, and loads between nine and eleven times their body weight occur when volleyball players land. (With years and years of experience taking care of the Philadelphia 76ers basketball team and the Pennsylvania Ballet, I have seen my share of jumper's knee. In fact, by midseason it is hard to find a pro basketball player who is not a little sore at the bottom tip of the kneecap.)

KNEEPAD

Young Adult Knee Conditions

Patellar Pain

Patellar Dislocation

Patellar Tendinitis ("Jumper's Knee")

Chondral Defect

Cartilage (Meniscus) Tear

Ligament Tear (especially ACL)

Stress Fracture

Interestingly, eccentric muscle training and exercise, along with a good stretching program, are the cornerstones of nonoperative treatment for jumper's knee and other "insertional tendinopathies" like Achilles tendinitis and tennis elbow. For those who don't respond to conservative measures—including things like shockwave therapy or plasma rich protein (PRP) injection—or other newer interventions, surgery can be very effective. (You might have noticed that I did not mention cortisone injection, and that is because cortisone is a no-no for the infrapatellar tendon, as it can cause a rupture of the tendon. Elsewhere in and around the knee, and for many other joints and tendons, cortisone is fine when used properly.)

From a diagnostic standpoint, the symptoms can be divided into four stages: Stage 1, when pain occurs only after activity; Stage 2, when pain is present at the beginning of an activity, dissipates after warmup, and then reappears after the activity; Stage 3, when pain occurs during and after activity, affecting performance; and Stage 4, when the tendon ruptures, causing a chronic weakness of the tendon.

Chondral Defect

Your knee cushion can suffer damage (what I refer to as a pothole, also called a chondral lesion) as a result of a severe fall, a traumatic sports injury, a previous injury, or simply being worn down over time. Interestingly, immobilization over a long period of time can also lead to cartilage damage—another strike against the use of casts and longer periods of immobilization, not to mention a sedentary lifestyle.

Potholes in articular cartilage can exist on their own, but they are sometimes accompanied by damage to ligaments and menisci. These defects come in all sizes and can be focal or diffuse. They can happen in otherwise healthy knees or in arthritic ones (called degenerative chondral defects in these latter cases). The bigger and deeper they are, the more of a problem they present. Sometimes, individuals with OCD (see page 16) can be without symptoms when they are younger and never know that they had this other condition lurking, and then as young adults they develop a large defect where the OCD lesion was.

KNEEPAD

I sometimes tell my patients, "I get all the jumpers." That's because I've taken care of some of the best "jumpers" in the world for many years—the Philadelphia 76ers basketball team and the Pennsylvania Ballet.

Cartilage "Meniscus" Tear

Traumatic injury and degenerative wear are the culprits for damage to the menisci. The most common event that leads to these tears is a twisting of the knee when the joint is in a bent position. Like the potholes just discussed, meniscus tears can also be seen in conjunction with damage to other parts of the knee.

Together with the swelling and pain that are common to other knee injuries, this condition is occasionally characterized by mechanical symptoms such as locking of the knee or the inability to straighten it because a renegade piece of meniscus impinges the joint mechanism. "Popping" or "clicking" is sometimes a symptom in these cases; many people just have localized discomfort on the inner or outer side of the joint.

Ligament Tear

This injury can certainly be seen on an MRI, but I (and any good sports doc) can tell on a quick physical exam if there is abnormal motion, laxity, or outright instability, and which exact ligament (or combination of ligaments) is torn.

Injured cruciate and collateral ligaments are considered "sprains" and are graded on a severity scale:

Anyone who has had a knee injury or surgery is at higher risk for cartilage damage because no matter how well you healed or how successful the procedure was, the mechanics of the joint can be altered.

Grade 1: The ligament is mildly damaged; it has been stretched a little, but is still tight and is able to help keep the knee joint stable. There is no significant laxity on exam.

Grade 2: The ligament is stretched to the point where it becomes somewhat loose, but it is still connected at both ends. (This is often referred to as a partial tear of the ligament.)

Grade 3: This sprain is commonly referred to as a complete tear of the ligament—the ligament has been pulled apart into two pieces, with shredding sometimes, too, and the knee joint has significant instability.

CRUCIATE LIGAMENTS

The **anterior cruciate ligament** (ACL) is also an important stabilizer, and if it's torn, you can have a "trick" knee that shifts and goes out during certain activities. Most people with ACL tears are able to go to the gym, jog, bike, or swim, but if they have to stop and start or change direction in sports like skiing, basketball, and tennis, the knee is more likely to go out on them.

The ACL can be injured in several ways:

- Rapid change of direction
- Sudden stop
- Sudden deceleration while running
- Landing incorrectly after a jump
- Hyperextension of the knee
- Direct contact or collision, such as a football tackle

When you injure your ACL, you might hear a "popping" noise and may feel your knee give out from under you. Other typical symptoms include:

- Pain accompanied by swelling (blood in the knee) within 24 hours. These initial symptoms may resolve on their own; however, if you return to sports, your knee will probably be unstable and you risk causing further damage to the menisci and articular cartilage.

- Loss of full range of motion
- Tenderness along the joint, especially in the back of the knee
- Discomfort while walking

Partial tears of the ACL are rare (they usually tear all the way), and more than half of all ACL injuries are accompanied by damage to other structures in the knee. Partial tears usually become complete over time, as the knee is still prone to problems that make further tearing likely.

Active individuals with ACL tears usually require surgery to stabilize the knee. Then they must participate in a stepwise rehabilitation program before getting back to sports and other higher-level activities. In addition, we now know that certain individuals are more predisposed to ACL tears and that preventive programs work, and should be mandatory for all young athletes (especially females) and for anyone who has had an ACL reconstruction. These latter individuals are more likely to re-tear not only the one that was surgically fixed, but also the opposite healthy one. (There will be more on this later, when we focus on knee exercise and injury prevention.)

The **posterior cruciate ligament** (PCL) can tear when the knee is bent and an object forcefully strikes the shin and pushes the upper tibia backwards, as happens in a car crash, which is why damage to the PCL is one type of "dashboard injury." The other common mechanism is a sports injury when an athlete suddenly hyperextends the knee. These situations stress the PCL, and if the force is high enough, a PCL tear will result.

The most common symptoms of a PCL tear are quite similar to those of an ACL tear: knee pain, swelling (usually much less than with the ACL tears, and sometimes even no swelling), and decreased motion. There may also be a sensation that the knee "popped" or gave out. Problems with instability in the weeks and months following PCL injury are not as common as instability following an ACL tear.

Most patients who have a PCL issue can do fine without surgery. When patients have instability after a PCL injury, they usually state that they can't "trust" their knee, or that something just doesn't feel right. If complaints persists, it may be an indicator that surgery is recommended.

COLLATERAL LIGAMENTS

The **medial collateral ligament** (MCL) is injured more often than the **lateral collateral ligament** (LCL) because you are much more likely to get struck on the outer side of the knee (think "clipping" in football).

Injuries to the collateral ligaments are usually caused by a force that pushes the knee sideways. (These are often contact injuries, but not always.) MCL (inner) tears occur as the result of a direct blow to the outside of the knee that forces it to buckle inward toward the other knee; blows to the inside of the knee that push the knee outward, away from the other knee, injure the outer LCL.

Collateral ligament tears are characterized by:

- Pain on the inside or outside of the knee

- Swelling over the site of the injury

- A limp

- Instability—the feeling that your knee is giving way

Stress Fracture

A small crack in a bone is another type of overuse injury that can occur around the knee area when the area is repetitively overloaded in ways that it is not used to handling and inadequate time is given to rest and recovery. It can also result if the intensity, duration, or frequency of an activity is increased too rapidly and the body does not have adequate time to adapt. If a patient reports this type of overuse history, and has focal tenderness over a bony area, then an MRI or bone scan can easily confirm the diagnosis of a stress fracture. X-rays should be done first, but because they are often negative, especially in the earlier stages (sometimes referred to as a stress reaction), an MRI should be ordered if a stress fracture is suspected.

The Mature Frame

We previously discussed how wear and tear starts to impact the knees in early adulthood, but age-related changes (none of them good) really kick in when we reach our late thirties and early forties. This is especially true if you are overweight, had a prior knee injury, or have a genetic predisposition that compromises your hinges in some way.

KNEEPAD

Sometimes there can be multiple ligaments torn at once. These are usually more serious injuries.

Decades of wear and tear significantly increase susceptibility to patellar pain syndromes (the undersurface of the kneecap begins to develop some arthritis-related softening, something extremely common but not always symptomatic) and to the soft tissue damage (tendinitis and tendinopathy) that we discussed previously. Middle-aged and older folks don't have to be sports and recreation fanatics to experience those woes because it doesn't take much to aggravate or tear a worn part; a person in this group can suffer an injury while gardening, bowling, or just getting out of the car. And when something breaks down or tears for this age group, it's not young, healthy tissue that we might be able to repair with a relatively simple procedure and relatively simple rehab; it's beat-up tissue that presents more of a therapeutic challenge. Also, the body's own healing capabilities are not what they used to be; healing takes longer and is not always complete.

Along with a full measure of those common knee woes that younger people get, mature folks get a couple that occur much more often with advancing years.

Osteoarthritis

Wear and tear is more and more of an issue with each year north of age 50 because there's no getting around the degeneration that any machine parts would have after more than half a century of operation.

On top of that, if you're overweight, you increase the possibility for and severity of arthritis. For every extra pound you carry, your knee thinks it's 5 to 7 pounds, so small amounts of weight gain are amplified across the knee—especially if it's unusually worn (as is seen in ex-athletes and weekend warriors); if you're bowlegged, knock-kneed, or have another genetic disposition that causes an alignment problem; or if you've had a previous injury.

Once you start getting arthritis, your knee lubricant (synovial fluid) becomes less viscous; instead of the "oil" it was, it becomes more like water, and you can feel a "grind" in your hinges as the surfaces get rougher and rougher and the lubrication and shock absorption systems begin to fail. Once those beautiful, smooth joint surfaces are violated and the

KNEEPAD

I recently had the great honor of working with baseball legend Hank Aaron on a national arthritis awareness campaign. "The Hammer" (still the home run king in my book) spent 23 years in the majors and was never on the disabled list. A few years after his retirement, he began to develop arthritis in his knee. This is true of many professional and high-level athletes later in their lives. I guess all those miles rounding the bases caught up with him. The arthritis began to interfere with his life, but with some simple measures, he was able to "get back in the game," get active again, and enjoy life. Hank instinctively knew the importance of motion, and that sedentary was not an option.

harder undersurfaces are exposed, it's very easy to suffer further damage. Add a little fuel to the fire—chronic inflammation—and that's how osteoarthritis progresses.

Knee arthritis can be mild, moderate, or severe, and, interestingly, symptoms don't always correlate with the severity of arthritis seen on x-rays or during arthroscopy. In fact, as I have learned from doing arthroscopy on thousands of knees, x-rays can often underestimate the degree of damage to the joint cushion or the degree of arthritis. Arthritic wear can involve the medial (inner) compartment, the lateral (outer) compartment, or the patella (patellofemoral joint). Sometimes it involves all three compartments; other times, just one or two. Isolated medial and/or patellar wear are both very common.

Patellar problems are no less of an issue in this group than they are in younger people, but they are less likely to fully resolve in this group because too much wear has all too often set in. Kneecap wear is very common, and it is a great example of a stealth problem that is just waiting to happen. As I've mentioned, it is one of those types of localized arthritis that is often without symptoms. Therefore, many adults don't know they have it until they sign up with an overzealous personal trainer or take the wrong fitness class. You're fine all along until something such as step aerobics loads the kneecap and all of a sudden, your knee is killing you, it's swollen, and you just found your weak link. Or you start running stadium steps (yes, some adults actually still do that), or you work with a personal trainer who is getting paid to get results and he or she pushes you really

hard with lots of squats and lunges. These exercises are great for building your legs and your butt, but they apply tremendous force under kneecaps that have weakened with age. There's nothing necessarily wrong with those programs if you have healthy knees, but kneecap wear is one of the most common problems I see in my kneecentric practice, and most problems are very preventable with proper workout design.

Sometimes, the kneecap is just fine and the arthritis is in the main part of the joint, medially, laterally, or both. These knees tend to better tolerate flexed knee activities like stairs, squats, lunges, and leg extensions, but hurt more in everyday standing and walking when the knee is loaded in a straighter position. The point to remember is that arthritis has many faces, and this is why treatment plans and exercise routines must be personalized. One size does not fit all.

Your hinges may have been a little creaky here and there, but they weren't really much of a problem until they were asked to do something they weren't in good-enough shape to do. Again, there's no real cure for arthritis, but there are plenty of things that your doctor *and* you can do to shape up. (Coming soon to a page in front of you.)

Baker's Cyst/Popliteal Cyst (and other fluid collections)

Whenever the knee is irritated, especially on a chronic repetitive basis, a fluid-filled sac, called a Baker's cyst, can form in the back of the knee (the popliteal area). This is an extremely common condition (I sometimes see 10 or 20 a week in my office), especially after age 40. Women are more likely than men to have one, and it can appear spontaneously in an otherwise normal knee. More often, they are associated with a meniscus tear or with arthritis. In the latter case, chronic inflammation creates excess synovial fluid in the knee that finds its way into small bursae in the back of the knee, filling up at times like a little water balloon.

Osteoarthritis, chondral defects, and meniscus tears are the primary instigators for fluid buildup in the knee. Baker's cysts may cause posterior knee pain and/or tightness behind the knee when it is flexed or extended, but they are not very tender and most people aren't aware that they have one unless it grows to a certain point (some are as large as a grapefruit!). As a rule, we don't operate on Baker's cysts because that can't be done through the scope (they actually form outside

JOINT DISCUSSION

My left kneecap is a real source of frustration for me. I often start a conversation with a new patient the same way. "Look, I have the same thing," I'll say as I bring the patient's hand to my knee. "You think your knee is bad, feel this," I continue as I introduce him or her to the "broken glass" sensation under my patella—it feels like there are Rice Krispies in there.

That knee is pretty bad, but believe it or not, I've never had an MRI done on it because I know what it would show. Patients always ask, "Can I get a new MRI?" because they think it will show something different. No, they can't. They've just flared up the same thing—osteoarthritis. The approach I recommend for them is the same one I prescribe for myself: keep my weight down, take joint supplements, exercise the extensor mechanism so it's strong and flexible, avoid those things (such as skiing, a former love) that I know are going to provoke my knee, and moderate the things I still love (tennis) that also provoke the knee.

the capsule of the knee joint and can't be seen or accessed through the scope), because the open procedure is complicated (cysts are usually located near the neurovascular bundle, a major artery and nerve), and because there is a 50 percent recurrence rate for them. So we just don't want to go digging around in there, with such a high failure rate, unless absolutely necessary. More conservative approaches—fluid extraction and sometimes arthroscopic repair of whatever is irritating the knee in the first place—will usually "tame" the cyst. (These cysts usually never go away completely, but you can often get them to behave better. The one exception is in children, who sometimes get a popliteal cyst, and they will often resolve on their own, and even disappear completely. Not so for adults.)

Other types of fluid collections include "Housemaid's Knee" (a bursa fluid collection in the front of the knee on top of the kneecap, from kneeling repetitively and irritating the front of the knee area), ganglion cysts (jelly-filled sacs that can form in or around the knee), and meniscal and/or synovial cysts. Fortunately, the overwhelming majority of cysts are benign and nothing to worry about, but all should be checked out (just like skin moles should be) to make sure there is not something more serious, such as a tumor (extremely rare but they do happen) going on in the knee.

KNEE REST

Before moving on to the next step, which addresses balky and damaged knees, allow me to address a couple of areas that will help you avoid injury and maximize the benefits of a knee-centric exercise program.

Posture

Loss of an erect frame is insidious in that decline is imperceptible as it progresses. Each incremental bend or slouch doesn't show up on our radar, but we get the (startling) picture one day when we catch ourselves in a mirror and the image doesn't jibe with the one we have in our memory. No matter how old you are, these simple tips are worth heeding:

- Sit up straight (as parents and teachers often harp): head erect and shoulders back
- Stand up straight: head erect, feet shoulder-width apart, shoulders in line with ankles
- Walk erect: head up, shoulders back
- Strengthen your core

KNEEPAD

Mature Knee Conditions

Patellar Pain

Tendinitis and Tendinopathy

Osteoarthritis

Chondral Defect

Degenerative Meniscus Tears

Ligament Tears

Baker's Cyst/Popliteal Cyst

Housemaid's Knee

Ganglion Cysts

De-Stress Your Knees

Prolonged sitting at work or when you travel can play havoc with your knees. Get up and move around for a couple of minutes every hour; if that's not possible, slide your feet or sway them back and forth while seated to keep your hinges oiled. Remember, *motion is lotion*, and as one of my very active elderly patients (who actually rode her bike to the hospital on the day she was to have her hip replaced) said, "If you rest, you rust."

"De-Sudden" Your Movement

Unless required for sport or self-preservation, abrupt twists, turns, starts, and stops should be avoided, especially if you are not used to them or not adequately warmed up, or not in shape.

Take a Load Off

Remind yourself often that your body is not a crane. When you pick up anything—free weight or feather—from the floor, bend at the knees, be square to the object, and balance it and yourself as you rise at a measured pace; when you walk with a heavy object, make sure the weight is held close to your body so it is transferred to your heels—not to your toes or midfeet.

KNEEPAD

To check your posture, stand as you naturally do, sideways in front of a mirror. If your shoulders extend beyond your buttocks, your back is too tight; if the middle of your back is out farther than your buttocks, you're slumping. Both conditions add unnecessary stress to your knees and your entire frame.

Brace Yourself

If you're rehabbing a knee or you have a "trick" one, there's no shame is using a "crutch" for it—an elastic wrap or one of the sturdier supports that are covered in depth in Step 6.

Rise Right

Joints, especially older ones, are stiffest first thing in the morning. Don't ask your knees to do their thing before they've had their coffee, so to speak. Again, no sudden movements upon awakening, and no strenuous activity before you've had a chance to limber them up a bit (another Step 4 topic).

RISK AND REWARD

Weak links, together with repetitive wear and tear, prey upon your knee components. Cartilage is damaged or lost and other soft tissue loses elasticity (just as old rubber

KNEEPAD

Your body is not a crane.

bands do), making your inherently unstable hinges more so. If you strengthen your weak links as best you can (three guesses about how that can be done would likely include exercise, wouldn't they?), you'll be as active as you can be.

Let me repeat: Sedentary is not an option.

And regular golf or tennis or aerobics or circuit training isn't enough, either. If you want to stay healthy or recover faster and more completely from knee injury and pain, there's no substitution for building up muscle and fine-tuning coordination with the comprehensive cross-training and support recommendations in these pages.

It's time to turn this one.

WOE IS KNEE

Knees are my game and I'm going to show you everything in the playbook about how they get injured and how they should be treated. Before we get to that—the "meat on the bones," so to speak—there are a couple of lessons to explore.

Dr. Joe Torg taught me many things during my training a long time ago, back when I was a kneeophyte, and one of the things I'll never forget was what he often said, tongue in cheek as usual, as he watched his excited orthopedic residents working with some fancy new instruments: "The arthroscope is the tool of the devil."

What he meant then is still true today: The arthroscope is so easy to use, it's prone to be overused. More than five million people visit orthopedic surgeons annually for knee problems, and we surgeons have to constantly be on guard against overuse and make sure we're using the scope for the right reasons, for the right results, on the right patient, and at the right time. All easier said than done.

That being said, the arthroscope is just an incredible tool that puts its stamp on most of the pages in this chapter. As I said earlier, it was used first on the knee, and now it's put into just about every joint. Elbows and shoulders are probed and repaired on a regular basis, and scopes are finding their way into ankles and hips. Some contemporary pioneers are even putting scopes into the spine.

Anything that's relatively easy for a doctor to do, patients are willing to have done, and arthroscopy is right up there in the top five most commonly performed surgical procedures. According to recent data, there are more than one million arthroscopic procedures done annually in the United States, and 85 percent involve the knee joint. It has lived up to its potential and it's perfect for those who are accustomed to fast and effective solutions, but it is not indicated for some of the patients who show up in my office looking for relief.

KNEE PAIN?

When your knee hurts, it's not always the knee. And any orthopedic surgeon worth his or her salt knows to listen to a patient's history first, and then be on the lookout for other possibilities during a comprehensive physical examination that follows.

This is especially true in younger and older folks whose source of pain may not necessarily be in the knee. Children who come to my office complaining that a knee hurts when they run, or just about all patients who have knee pain, have to have the hips checked because of the way the nervous system and its high-speed cables, the nerves, work. The nerve that motorizes the hip is also the one that brings sensation to the knee area, and some pediatric and adult hip conditions can cause "referred" knee pain. The key point is that in most knee pain cases, your doctor should take your hip through a quick range-of-motion test as part of the clinical exam.

Many in the older crowd have arthritis to one degree or another in the knee that causes intermittent or constant pain. But because there is no cure for arthritis, and very few options to improve this condition with an arthroscope, addressing knee pain in these cases is more about a combination of lifestyle approaches, especially weight loss. Multiple interventions include (surprise-surprise) exercise because a weak thigh is one of the risk factors for osteoarthritis. That's not to say that a scope is completely out of the question, but the more advanced your arthritis is, the less likely a scope will offer significant lasting relief. Talk to your surgeon about this very issue and you won't be one of the many disappointed folks who go through a knee scope

JOINT DISCUSSION

Knee pain in some preschool and early elementary school children is related to hip pathology. In general, I check the hip, and the first thing I do after having a patient lie down is flex the affected knee and observe how the hip moves. Just as lower back problems can cause pain to the front of the thigh and the knee, out-of-whack hips can send symptoms down the line.

only to be told a few months later that they need a knee replacement.

Getting back to that important quad muscle, people who have arthritis get pulled into a vicious cycle: The knee is swollen and/or hurting and/or stiff, so people sit down every chance they get and lean on banisters, compensating any way they can, and the knee isn't used as much as it should be; muscle strength and mass diminish, weakening the critical support structure; the knee still hurts, is used less and less, and becomes more and more vulnerable to pain and even further injury. Fortunately, there are some things in our armamentarium, discussed below, that can stop this downhill spiral.

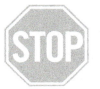

There are a couple of pain-causing conditions that demand immediate medical and surgical intervention. If you have one of these, it's a red flag and don't be surprised if you find yourself in the operating room without passing Go.

Locked Knee

One moment you're fine, the next you can't straighten your knee. This is not a case when

An arthritic knee must be exercised, but it must be done the right way because high-impact loading will cause further damage to those cushions we discussed in Step 1. Running is definitely out, and most patients will have to compromise in some way (as I did when I put my skis away, and started playing more doubles than singles tennis). Remember, stopping activity completely is just not an option.

the knee "catches," or hangs up momentarily (as mine does on occasion,) after long periods of sitting. Gentle coaxing usually does the trick in those cases. It's a whole other kettle of fish if you've got a locked knee—it's mechanically jammed and it won't recover no matter what you try, although sometimes it will magically unlock on its own or after you put it through some maneuvers. You can expect to wind up with a scope in your knee posthaste to find out if a piece of cartilage flipped on itself or if a floating chip, also known as a loose body, is in the way (picture a door opening that has something wedged between the frame and the door, and needs to be removed if you expect the door to properly close again).

Bloody Fluid

Extracting some fluid from the knee is part of a comprehensive diagnostic workup for many knee problems. Normal fluid is yellowish like apple juice; if there's blood in it, something significant is going on: a torn ACL, a torn meniscus, or a chondral fracture. You probably will wind up with a scope in your knee at some point.

Cloudy Fluid

This could be caused by a variety of systemic (i.e., an underlying medical problem throughout the body) rheumatology problems, such as rheumatoid arthritis, lupus, or

An infected knee, accompanied by fever, is an absolute emergency.

Lyme disease, or septic arthritis caused by a bacterial infection. (Anyone can get septic arthritis, and it is not uncommon in children.) If you're lucky, your cloudy fluid will "only" be the result of gout or its distant relative, pseudogout, both of which become more common in adults (especially men) with each passing year. An infection requires surgery on an urgent basis. Other causes of cloudy fluid can usually be managed medically, without the need for surgery.

Complete Knee Dislocation

With significant trauma, like an auto or motorcycle crash, or even a very hard hit to the knee in football, the knee can be severely twisted, tearing not only multiple ligaments but also injuring the major artery and vein housed in the popliteal fossa just behind the knee joint. Nerve damage can also occur. This is a major emergency that will require not only an orthopedic surgeon but also a vascular surgery specialist. Although this type of injury is not very common, one must be on the alert any time there has been severe trauma to the knee. The clock is ticking when these major nerves and blood vessels are injured, and permanent damage can occur if there is a delay in diagnosis and treatment.

JOINT DISCUSSION

I've really got to put on my thinking cap and use all my detective skills when I extract cloudy fluid from a knee. It means an infection may be afoot, and that's something you can't sit on—it has to be taken care of *that day*. So I give my diagnostic skills a thorough workout until I get to the bottom of what is "clouding" the picture. Then I'll know what the next step should be to clear things up. Fortunately, all cases of cloudy fluid are not from an infection.

FIRST AID

Of course, if there is severe swelling, or a limp, or loss of range of motion, or fever and chills associated with knee pain, get to the doc pronto. Many common knee woes, however, do not require a doctor visit because swelling and pain diminish, and functionality improves, shortly after an episode occurs. Unfortunately, the first inclination most people have at any point of a knee condition that doesn't require immediate attention is to baby it. They'll keep it elevated, take some pills, use some heat or ice, and, worst of all, compensate for it when they walk or climb stairs. As a result, inflammation sticks around longer than it has to, stiffness is more than it should be, and thigh and calf muscles (part of the knee support system) get out of shape. By all means, employ common sense about the need to see a doctor and be careful when you have a knee woe, but what is true for back ailments is true here: In most cases, the sooner you move it, the sooner you heal it.

If your symptoms subside and your knee is stable, first aid, followed by low-impact exercise, may be all you need. The RICE protocol is effective for most orthopedic injuries.

Rest: Take a break from the activity that caused the injury.

Ice: Use cold packs for 20 minutes at a time, several times a day. *Do not apply ice directly to the skin.* (This is especially true for freezer gel packs that will get as cold as your freezer is set and that could cause frostbite on the skin. I prefer a thin wash cloth moistened with cool water and wrung out, with the ice or gel pack over that and held in place with an elastic wrap. A bag of frozen peas or corn can also work nicely, but don't eat them after you've thawed and refrozen them.) It is important to note that ice therapy doesn't have to be a chore; you can often apply the ice pack, hold it in place with an Ace wrap, and be up and about.

- Compression: To prevent additional swelling, wear an elastic compression bandage. *Do not wrap too tightly.*

- Elevation: *This is the most important component.* To prevent or reduce swelling, recline when you rest, and put your leg up higher than your head or your heart. Propping it up on an ottoman, lower than the level of your heart, can still allow significant swelling to occur.

In addition to the RICE protocol, nonsteroidal anti-inflammatory drugs (NSAIDs) such as aspirin and ibuprofen reduce pain and swelling. For pro athletes, we have other tricks to minimize downtime and accelerate recovery. (More on this later.)

Once your condition is under control, the Recovery exercises in Step 5 will reduce the time it takes to move from woe to "go," and minimize your susceptibility to a relapse. However, if your condition doesn't improve after a few days, get thee to an orthopedist's office and he or she will take it from there.

THE INCREDIBLE ARTHROSCOPE

As most of you know (and as we will soon explore in depth), the scope has evolved into a tremendous treatment tool for a host of medical complaints, but I'll remind you that it started out as just a diagnostic tool. Then came the probe, akin to the picks that dentists use to check for cavities; they don't just look, they feel around the tooth structures to determine how tight they are and whether they're moving properly in the jawbone. We did a whole lot of "looking" and "feeling around" in the knee in the early days because the procedure was still primitive and awkward. That is no longer the case, and the technological advances made knee procedures easier to do and recover from, and more effective, too. So we surgeons routinely snip, cut, attach, and pave away to restore knee function. Short of knee replacements, we are now doing almost everything through the scope.

I will admit that replacing torn ligaments with new tissue and filling those potholes in articular cartilage is pretty sexy, but the scope is still every bit the fantastic diagnostic tool that it started out to be. It is still the most accurate way of knowing what's going on in a knee before the really cool stuff starts.

MRIs have come on the scene and usually provide a fairly precise diagnosis. They're great at showing the meniscus and ligaments, and for providing views of cysts and stress fractures, but they just don't provide definitive images yet of the knee cushion (articular cartilage) that would identify an early stage of damage, the size of defects, and whether the cartilage is amenable to regeneration. Some newer MRI technology does allow better joint cushion qualitative and quantitative analysis that can allow for health assessment of the cushion, but these MRI scanners are not readily available everywhere. When they are, I'm certain they will not only help with research endeavors, but will also influence how and when we treat certain knee conditions.

I tell my patients that the MRI is 95 percent accurate (and I'd love to find a weatherman anywhere close to that), but as tremendous as that record is, it still means that something is missed in 1 out of every 20 cases. Those are usually the ones where the patient has not gotten any better after conservative treatment; the history, physical exam, and MRI just didn't add up to a satisfactory solution. The only way I can solve the puzzle and know for sure what the next step should be is to go in there for a look-see.

Today, we do a lot more than looking. We have very sophisticated instruments that are used with the scope for almost every type of knee procedure that you might need. I don't have to bend over and peek through the scope anymore because now I attach a miniature camera to the end of the scope and watch everything on a high-def flat screen that is right in front of me. I can zoom in if I want, brighten or darken an area to see it better, pan across the joint, videotape everything, and shoot high-def photos of whatever I want. There are better fixation devices for ligaments, including bioabsorbable screws (no more metal in the knee that shows up on an x-ray or the new airport scanners), and bioabsorbable tacks to repair, rather than remove, torn menisci. We also have all sorts of arthroscopic drills, burrs, and picks—sometimes I feel like I'm at Home Depot! I'm telling you, it's night and day what has happened with the technology since the early days.

As incredible as the arthroscope is, however, we still can't cure everything with it. Sometimes we look around, using it as the

JOINT DISCUSSION

In the old days, that exciting time when the arthroscope was first used, I actually had to bend over and peek into the end of a long tube like I would if I were using a microscope or telescope. My assistant would hold the leg and have no visual clue as to what I was seeing through the peephole; it was what we call triangulating, putting instruments and the scope into different sides of the knee and having them find themselves at the right spot in the joint.

Triangulation is a skill that is still very hard to develop, even though we now use large monitors and other innovations in the procedure. We surgeons tend to take it for granted because we just get so good at it, but I'm always reminded to be patient when I train young residents and see them struggle to even find an instrument in the knee, let alone be able to use it for sophisticated surgery.

incredible diagnostic tool it still is, and find arthritis or another condition that is beyond the scope's capability right now. This news doesn't square with the usual patient expectation that we can fix anything. I think we're

doing tremendous work right now and that the future is very bright because of some amazing things on the horizon, but facts are facts. Patient expectations have never been higher, and that's where you need a surgeon who will take the time to paint an honest picture for you. Expectations fuel outcomes, so the more patients understand and reasonably expect going in to surgery, the happier they will be afterward. I see so many disappointed patients who come to me for a second opinion after having surgery elsewhere. The usual problem is not that anything was done improperly, but rather that realistic expectations were not set by the surgeon.

PRIOR TO SURGERY

Most things going on in knees can be addressed with the scope. We're about to get to them, but you should know a thing or two that I discuss with all of my patients before they lie down on the operating table.

Realistic expectations and the need for compliance with a rehab program are right up front after I complete my examination. Yes, medicine generally, and arthroscopy specifically, are miraculous in many respects, but there are some critical factors that influence surgical outcomes.

The success of your surgery will often be determined by the degree of injury or damage in your knee. For example, if you damage your knee and the smooth articular cushion has worn away completely, then full recovery may not be possible. You may be advised to find a low-impact alternative form of exercise.

College or professional athletes who have the same injury as you do have better prospects for complete recovery because of highly developed support muscles and conditioning programs. They are also goal oriented and highly motivated to do all the necessary work for optimal recovery. And they heal quicker and more fully.

Physical therapy and exercise play a critical role in your final outcome.

A return to intense physical activity should only be done under the direction of your surgeon. It is usually a stepwise progression, like advancing to the next level in a video game.

Each surgery has a different recovery timetable based on exactly what was done. For simple arthroscopic procedures, it is reasonable to expect that within 6 to 8 weeks you should be able to engage in most of your former physical activities. Bigger surgeries, such as ACL reconstruction, can require 6 to 8 months before full sports activity is allowed. The patient feels great much sooner than that, but the new graft takes time to become part of your body and to gain sufficient strength to allow high-level sports and activities.

For all surgeries, the better shape you are in going into it, the quicker your recovery will usually be. (Another reason to remain fit year-round!)

JOINT DISCUSSION

When I would assist Dr. Torg with knee surgeries during my training, I'd catch his playful eyes and could tell he was sporting that signature half grin under his mask. It was the same grin that he displayed often in an office setting where he put things just so for a student. "Knees are just like faces," he said on more than one occasion. "Each one is a little different."

How right he was. I've scoped thousands of knees and can't take any for granted. Each patient, and each knee, is unique, and must be treated as such.

If your job involves heavy work, such as construction labor, you may require more time to return to your job than if you have a sedentary job.

Now that we've dispensed with the preliminaries, let's "cut" into the main course.

COMMON KNEE COMPLAINTS AND TREATMENTS

We see all different kinds of wear patterns in the knee, just like we do on car tires or the soles of shoes. If all three cushions go, it's a tricompartment case, the most challenging of all. That's when the subject of a knee replacement comes to the fore, but there is much more we can do for you before that point is reached.

Patellar Pain

I know I've talked a lot about the patella, but kneecap issues are one of the most common knee problems I see in my practice day in and day out. They are also one of the most frustrating to manage, and this is where more knowledge and understanding go a long way. The patients who take the time to understand the issue do far better than those who just go doctor-hopping for a quick fix.

The results of patella surgery for people who have chronic kneecap pain or kneecap issues

are just not that great. As I mentioned before, I tell my patients (especially the teens and their parents) that it's sort of like a migraine headache—it's painful and disabling, but a brain x-ray is going to be normal, a brain scan is going to be normal, an EEG will be normal, and just as brain surgery is not used for migraine headaches, knee surgery offers no magic for most cases of patellar pain. So an invasive procedure usually isn't going to cure it.

Although most patients who have patellar pain expect it to be operated on, I tell them a conservative approach is usually the best way to go. They mistakenly think that the severity of their symptoms means that it must be a serious and surgical condition. This is not always the case in orthopedics, or in medicine in general for that matter. One can have cancer with absolutely no symptoms, or have a relatively minor problem that drives one crazy in terms of unrelenting symptoms. So it is with achy kneecaps.

A conservative approach is also used sometimes in cases that have visible evidence of kneecap damage or instability. NSAIDs, Tylenol, a sleeve or special patellar brace, avoidance of competitive sports and intense exercise, and physical therapy might do the trick even in some of the more serious cases.

If problems persist or the joint does not return to normal function after months and months of proper conservative care, we can always go in with the scope to better evaluate the situation. If the kneecap is riding off track, we can do a lateral release: pull the kneecap over, tighten up on one side, and let the seam out on the other side, so to speak. Again, the prospects aren't great for this procedure, but some people need it. Sometimes, I'll find a chondral defect that needs treatment, or some loose bodies or floating chips to remove. Some patients have a painful plica band adjacent to the kneecap (a band of tissue that is left over when the knee was formed)

JOINT DISCUSSION

Osgood-Schlatter Disease used to be treated with surgery followed by a cast to immobilize the area. That not only made a lot of children (and their parents) miserable, it didn't work well enough to justify all the trouble, so we take a totally different approach today.

Modern OSD case management involves slowing an active child down a bit, use of RICE, a special brace, and a lot of stretching and targeted strengthening.

The "slowing" part is no easier today than it was in the past, but it can be managed. Typically, a child affected by OSD plays on multiple sports teams. My goal isn't to have him or her drop a favorite activity; instead, it's to eliminate duplication of exercise that aggravates the condition. For example, if a child runs laps to train for one sport, he or she shouldn't do them later that day or the next day for another sport. So I tell my young patient-athletes to have a frank talk with all of their coaches about what it will take for them to keep playing. It is often more about turning down the volume than about switching the station. This is true for most overuse injuries.

that causes irritation. It's removed very easily through the scope for an instant cure that sure is rewarding. However, most people have one of these bands and, as it is with the appendix, it doesn't have to be removed unless a problem (usually pronounced focal pain just on the medial or inner edge of the kneecap) can be traced directly to it—and that just isn't so in many cases.

Patellar Tendinitis and Tendinopathy

Tendinitis implies inflammation of the tendon, which is often seen in more acute cases of jumper's knee. However, as things become recurrent and more chronic, the tendon shows less and less inflammation and more signs of internal damage, a type of avascular (and thus limited ability to heal) scar tissue, which we call tendinopathy.

Microtears to the patellar tendon often exceed the body's ability to heal the area unless the aggravating activity is stopped for a sufficient amount of time. Therefore, most patients with jumper's knee are treated conservatively, with the addition of quadriceps strengthening (especially eccentric) and stretching. Some patients do well with a neoprene knee sleeve or a band (Cho-Pat) that goes just below the kneecap. Patients with chronic jumper's knee

that does not respond to conservative care will need outpatient open surgery, which can be done with a small incision, to remove unhealthy tendon tissue. The operation is fairly simple, with good results, but the recovery and rehab is long, taking up to 6 months before a return to full activities is possible.

If the condition doesn't improve over time (up to a year is appropriate in most cases), there are a couple of procedures before open surgery has to be considered that might help a patient whose tendon symptoms are debilitating.

- Coblation microtenotomy: This minimally-invasive surgery uses radio waves to promote the growth of blood vessels in and around the tendon,which encourage repair and remodeling of damaged tissue.

- Extracorporeal Shock Wave Therapy (ESWT): This is a relatively new procedure that doesn't require an incision. Stimulation is transmitted through the skin via low-energy waves (little or no pain) over three-plus visits or via high-energy waves (requiring anesthesia) in one visit.

- Plasma Rich Protein: Many patients are having plasma rich protein, or PRP, injected into damaged tendons. The theory is that stem cells in this plasma (taken from your own blood) can jump-start the healing process and help to re-form more normal tendon tissue. Research results have been mixed, and the final verdict is not in yet. I do believe that this will have some role in the repair and regeneration of a variety of injuries in the future.

Some patients will completely rupture their infrapatellar tendon, and this requires relatively urgent surgery to reattach the torn ends. The same goes for those who rupture the quadriceps tendon just above the kneecap, something more common in middle-aged men and people with diabetes.

As always, the best treatment is prevention. For serious athletes who have jumper's knee, preseason conditioning should concentrate on a gradual increase in repetitive eccentric quadriceps contraction so that the patellar tendon can withstand repetitive loading. Proper warmup and stretching are essential, too. As for the rest of us, the programs in Step 5 will go a long way to keeping tendon problems at bay.

Arthritis

Along with patellar pain, this is the most common complaint I see. It is one that is often complicated by a patient's expectations of surgery after seeing a general practitioner who ordered an MRI and informed the patient that he or she has a torn meniscus. The patient shows up and tells me that the GP sent them to me for surgery that will solve all knee problems. Boy, I sure wish it was that easy. After all, I love doing arthroscopies, but as I have said before, that just isn't enough to schedule one right away, especially if the patient is over 50 years old and arthritis is a factor in play.

Yes, the knee hurts like hell and, yes, the scope can take care of the meniscus, but that may not help at all because the pain may be caused more by arthritis than by a "hanging chad" in the joint.

You'll recall that a distinction was made earlier between two types of cartilage. When it comes to articular cartilage, your cushion, you can have focal disrepair (chondral defects, those potholes I mentioned) or you can have more advanced damage, and that's what arthritis is. It can be localized or diffuse throughout the knee; wherever it is, there is increased friction (those Rice Krispies grinding behind my kneecap) and that increases inflammation and further cell damage. It's the vicious cycle, another pet topic of mine that I expound upon in Step 6.

JOINT DISCUSSION

This happens to me a dozen times a week: A patient comes in with an MRI in hand and expectations of a quick fix with the scope in mind.

"Not so fast," I say. "You've got a tear in the meniscus, but let's get a standing x-ray."

"Why do I need an x-ray?" the patient sighs. "Doesn't the MRI show you everything?"

"Nope."

I go on to tell him an MRI is terrific, but an x-ray adds a whole lot more to the clinical picture. It actually shows the degree of joint space narrowing, and the degree of arthritis, better than an MRI. If it's bone-on-bone, I can fix the meniscus, but that won't do much for the arthritis that has as much, if not a lot more, to do with the knee pain that was responsible for the visit.

The conversation continues with the x-ray in the light box. "Did the doctor tell you that you have advanced arthritis in your knee?" I ask.

"He said it was probably a little worn, but that I'd be fine after the surgery."

"Look," I say as I point to the x-ray. "You've lost a lot of cartilage, and the bones are a lot closer than they should be. Half or more of your pain is coming from arthritis. I can do something about that meniscus, but I can't promise you that everything will be completely resolved."

At that point, the patient is usually crestfallen, but there is no getting around the facts of his case, and we just have to be on the same page if we are to be successful going forward. "Don't expect a home run after the scope," I continue. "We can hit a single or a double and make you a little better, but you will still have to contend with the arthritis. You're going to have to lose some weight and take some supplements religiously, and we might have to try some injections using cortisone or viscosupplementation. And no matter what we do, a total knee replacement might be in your future. I'm hoping to buy you some time." And that's if the patient is lucky, and the arthritis is not too bad. For others with more advanced arthritis, a scope is out of the question and we are on to Plan B.

This isn't what the patient wanted to hear. No way. But it's the truth, and sometimes I can't win no matter how much I try to explain it. The patient came in with certain expectations, and he'll hobble out in search of another doctor who will tell him what he wants to hear.

We surgeons always talk about outcomes, but I think outcomes are not just how good you are technically, it's not how pretty the x-ray looks or how well the knee moves after the procedure—it's how the patient *feels* then. When it comes to surgery, it takes two to tango. So I have to make the right diagnosis and give the patient the straight scoop, so he or she can dance as best as possible.

Your cushion wears down over time because you aren't going to stop moving. Put a couple of dents or chips in articular cartilage, that opaque ball, or shave it over time as a result of wear and tear, and that explains a whole lot of knee symptoms I confront. You go from mild articular degeneration . . . to moderate . . . to gone. That's when you have the most advanced arthritis you can get; your patella and femur or femur and tibia are bone-on-bone, a condition that is never good but especially problematic when it's the bones composing the main joint you walk on every day. Talk about friction!

I'll hear the patient out, but then I'll do a thorough examination that includes a standing AP (anteroposterior, front-to-back) x-ray of both knees because the information they provide is indispensable in knee pain cases. Special views are also needed in many cases. Before I consider cutting into the joint I want to know about bone alignment, bone quality, soft tissue swelling, and bone spacing (or, put another way, how much cartilage has been lost), which is critical. If advanced arthritis is the main issue, then the scope shouldn't be used unless a loose body or tear is also causing some really significant mechanical impingement.

There are some docs who still think arthritis can be fixed with a scope, but it just can't

KNEEPAD

"Tweeners"

I have many patients who, because of their degree of arthritis, are beyond where I can help them with a scope; but they are not yet where they need or want a knee replacement. I call them tweeners, and there's no shortage of them. We certainly could use more stepwise surgical procedures or other new treatments for arthritis because it is a huge leap from a simple scope to a major joint replacement.

be done in the vast majority of cases. I'm not saying never because there are instances when the scope can improve the condition and I do it myself, but the more arthritis is the factor, the less the scope is going to be the answer. As a result, I find that I'm talking a lot of patients out of arthroscopy when arthritis is the main culprit.

It's also not a uniform thing that if you have arthritis, it's going to hurt, or if your knee is hurting, you're going to need a knee replacement. I even have a few patients who are bone-on-bone or very close to it, but believe it or not, they're asymptomatic. For the rest of us who are hurting because of this condition, and are not yet ready for knee replacement, there are still many things to offer.

■ Weight loss, if applicable (and it often is)

■ Supplements (see "Over-the-Counter Supplement Remedies for Arthritis" for specifics)

■ Injections:

- Cortisone: It's not long-acting, so I'll use it if somebody has a bad flare-up, or is going away or has a special occasion and they want to feel better for a week or two; in general, this shouldn't be introduced into a joint more than three times a year because too much exposure can be damaging to the joint. Think of it as a fire extinguisher, but not a longer-term solution.

- Viscosupplementation: Formulated from a natural substance that is similar to synovial fluid, a single injection (Synvisc-One) can last, in my experience, for anywhere from 6 (that is the claim listed on the Synvisc label) to 18 months. It is very safe, and it works at all stages of arthritis (although it is more effective early on). I use it so that patients can exercise comfortably to lose weight and to train support structures, which leads to more permanent relief when the injection wears off. Think of it as a longer-term solution for arthritis pain. Also, some recent research suggests that Synvisc-One may protect damaged or worn articular cartilage from further wear, something we call chondroprotection.

Once again, inflammation is your enemy. The really good news is that breakthroughs have been made related to blood biomarkers that allow us to predict and prevent joint wear. Also, new, high-resolution, 3-D-type qualitative MRI technology now gives doctors a chance to see joints at the metabolic level,

JOINT DISCUSSION

There was a very brave surgeon who did a controlled study involving two groups of patients who had arthritic knees. For one group, he went in with a scope and cleaned things up, and for the other, he made the little puncture holes and put stitches in as if the scope was done, but he actually didn't do any surgery within the knee at all. He evaluated all of the patients 6 months later in terms of how their knees felt, and discovered that whether they had the clean out procedure or the sham operation, the results were the same.

His research sure opened some eyes. We surgeons think we'll help these people who have arthritis, and, sure, they come back a month later and say they feel better. That's no doubt because the joint was flushed out and we slowed the patient down for a couple of weeks. But the net effect wouldn't be any better than if we had administered a placebo that enlists the mind in a cure.

Don't get me wrong, there are still some select patients with arthritis who can benefit from arthroscopy, but that requires an experienced, honest surgeon who not only looks at the MRI result, but also at special standing x-rays to determine the true degree of degeneration.

which enables us to catch joint surface damage and arthritis at a much earlier stage. But no matter what stage you're in, do everything in your power to keep it at bay: Lose weight, eat right, take supplements, and (oh no, not again) exercise to improve your prospects for staying active.

Chondral Defect

A cushion issue could be confined to just one side (compartment) of the tibiofemoral joint, or it could affect both compartments. Bow-legged individuals have worn cartilage on the medial, or inside, part of the knee; knock-kneed folks have a problem in their lateral, or outer, compartment. Excess irritation could also start in the patellofemoral joint, as it did in my case, and spread until it affects adjacent compartments. Sometimes damage can be very localized.

If I find loose chips in the knee, I have to look very hard for the source of those chips,

KNEEPAD

Over-the-Counter Supplement Remedies for Arthritis

- **Cosamin DS**, a glucosamine and chondroitin sulfate formulation from Nutamax Labs that also has manganese and ascorbate (vitamin C)

- **Cosamin ASU** (Avocado-Soybean Unsaponifiables), also from Nutramax, that includes glucosamine, chondroitin sulfate, and green tea extract

- **Zyflamend**, from New Chapter Organics, a combination of natural anti-inflammatory agents

- **Limbrel**, a flavocoxid, anti-inflammatory, and antioxidant ("medical food" category that requires a prescription)

- **Pycnogenol** (PCO), also available in pine bark or grapeseed extracts

- **Green tea extract**

- **Ginger**

- **Turmeric**

- **L-arginine**

- **Cayenne pepper**

- **Salicin** (willow bark)

- **Acetyl-L-carnitine**

- **Gamma linolenic acid** (GLA)

- **Branched-chain amino acids** (BCAA)

- **Coenzyme Q$_{10}$**

- **Omega-3s**

- **Flaxseed**

---

and I'll usually find a pothole (chondral defect) that is affecting the cushion and the bones of the knee. Until recently, the best way to repair the damage was to use the microfracture procedure that was pioneered by Dr. Richard Steadman, whereby special awls are used to puncture the crater and create scar tissue that fills the cavity via your body's own stem cells. This helps many patients, but there are concerns about the long-term durability of the repair tissue that forms.

Specialists now have an alternative way to "resurface" damaged knee cartilage: autologous chondrocyte implantation, or ACI. Healthy cartilage cells—the chondrocytes—are harvested from the patient during a simple

JOINT DISCUSSION

If you have an arthritic patellofemoral joint like I have, high-impact loading is not a good idea. Swimming is good, walking is good, but playing tennis as hard as I do is probably not the smartest thing. But I absolutely love it, so if there's a similar activity you'd rather not live without, weigh the plusses and minuses in your own head and go for it if the positive tips the scale in your favor—but only after you've done your preventive work to the max.

arthroscopic procedure, grown in culture in a lab, and then reimplanted during a second procedure into the damaged area where they grow into healthy new cartilage tissue. The cells, more than 12 million new chondrocytes, are in a liquid suspension no larger than a thimble. They'd spill out of the pothole if they were just squirted in, so the surgeon has to steal a bit of periosteum (fibrous membrane that covers bone) from the shin to use as a patch to cover the new chondrocytes. The patch is carefully sutured to the surface and then sealed with adhesive, like a blowout patch on a tire.

Nearly 9 in 10 patients experience good results with the ACI procedure, but it's an open operation requiring more complex techniques and more involved rehabilitation than an arthroscopy does (see page 36). ACI is usually performed on younger patients, who have better healing capability and will be able to benefit for a long time. Even though it's a bigger procedure, patients usually feel great after the surgery, but they must be on crutches for about 6 weeks because if they walk on the new cells right away, the cells will likely be destroyed before they have a chance to become part of the surrounding tissue. The initial post-procedure physical therapy includes a special machine that produces continuous passive motion (CPM) to rock the knee, like a baby in a cradle. It usually takes 9-plus months before any sports are allowed, depending on location and size of the defect, and the patient's commitment to their post-operative rehabilitation program.

KNEEPAD

Dr. Robert Salter, a visionary in Canada, discovered that motion enhanced the healing of articular cartilage, so continuous passive motion (CPM) is used after ACI and other cartilage regeneration procedures.

Meniscus Injuries

Meniscal tears are very common and probably the number-one reason for an arthroscopic knee procedure. Tears are usually removed, but can sometimes be saved or repaired: When people say they got a tear fixed, most of the time it was a relatively minor procedure whereby the surgeon removed (rather than *repaired*) a hanging shard of the meniscus that was flipping and flapping around and then the void was sculpted as best as possible to lessen friction between moving parts. (It's like when you have a hangnail—you don't remove the whole nail, you clip and file and preserve as much of the original structure as you can.)

In addition to a patient's age, where the meniscus damage is located impacts the success of a procedure. Tears in the "red zone," the outer edge that is closest to the blood supply, have the best prospects for total repair, especially in younger patients. There's also a red/white zone where there might be some blood supply to help healing; it's about 3 millimeters wide and it bridges the red zone with the white zone, which lacks any blood supply at all. Tears in this latter area, regardless of someone's age, can't be fixed yet. (However, there are exciting things on the horizon that are covered in the Afterword.) If the meniscus is repaired, it is a longer recovery than if a portion was just removed. This is because the meniscus is a very slow healing tissue.

We do everything we can to fully repair a red zone tear, from stitches to sculpting to injection of cellular growth factors. My friend and colleague Dr. Richard Steadman has even developed a scaffold that can be inlaid to promote healing and regeneration; it is stitched into the remaining meniscus, and then your body repopulates it over time with new tissue there. I can envision it being a big part of the future for knees, and even for shoulders.

If the meniscus is too damaged and has to be entirely removed, we know that significant arthritis will develop within 10 years or so. There's a procedure that isn't done often— mostly for younger patients who have a longer future to be concerned about—whereby cadaver tissue (a meniscal allograft) is transplanted using the scope.

After meniscal repair, even when conditions are perfect and the procedure is perfectly executed, there's still a re-tear or nonhealing rate of about 15 percent, especially in younger patients who aren't very "patient" about waiting to get back into the game. It doesn't make me the most popular guy around, but I have to

JOINT DISCUSSION

When I was in my training, surgeons would open the knee up with a big incision and be proud about how much meniscus they were able to remove, just as someone would brag about the size of a fish caught out in the ocean. Now we do all of the work through the scope, and we do everything we can to spare as much of the meniscus as possible because it's an important stabilizer of the knee and it's critical for shock absorption.

be the voice of reason in these cases because there's just no way around the 4-plus months that are necessary when a meniscus is stitched and saved (i.e., *repaired* not *removed*) before competitive activity can resume. Too often I hear, "Oh, can't you just take it out, doc?" No, I can't. I'm always focused on the best long-term outcome.

Cruciate Ligament Tears

Anterior cruciate ligament tears are a major issue, and we're seeing more and more complete tears (i.e., Grade 3 sprains) and doing more and more surgeries, probably because there are so many girls getting tears and there are more Baby Boomers who want to stay active after an ACL injury. The good news is they can opt for surgery at almost any time, as opposed to when I finished my training in 1982. The feeling then was if you're 40 and you've torn your ACL, you have to live with a loose knee and/or knee pain for the rest of your life. If a patient was 40 or older, we wouldn't think of fixing the ACL. Now, I've actually done a couple of 60-year-olds.

We employ the ACL reconstruction procedure that is quite common now. Whether you use your own tissue (an autograph) or donor tissue (an allograft) to restore your ACL, the procedure is done with incisions that are no more than 1 inch across. The knee isn't opened; a small incision is made high up on the shin bone, a little tunnel is created into the knee, and the rest of the work is done through the scope so we don't violate the knee any more than is absolutely necessary.

There's a variety of ways to get the new ligament to hold on, but the one that I use is bioabsorbable screws. Instead of being made of metal, they're made of hard plasticlike material that dissolves over time. I attach the ligament through the tunnel, and over time, your body grabs on to the tendon, the tendon gets its own blood supply, and the tissue actually remodels and becomes part of you.

JOINT DISCUSSION

Years ago, if you were 40 and you blew out your ACL, you would get a brace, and only if the knee was going out all the time would we put you through a surgery. Recently, a 60-year-old guy came into my office and told me he tore his ACL and wanted it repaired.

"I always spend the winter out in Colorado skiing black diamonds and double diamonds," he began, "and for 20 years I've had to put up with a torn ACL in the other knee. They told me I was too old to have it done." It was a story I've heard a thousand times. "I've struggled with that one my whole life. I've had to wear a brace; I've had to nurse it along. It really changed my enjoyment of skiing, and I won't go through that with this one. I want at least one good knee."

Age didn't matter to him, and as I listened to him further, I thought he was really on to something. What he said was quite insightful; it has stuck with me ever since, and it captures how much has changed in terms of how we treat things now in different age groups. "Twenty years ago, I was too old for an ACL reconstruction," he continued, "but now I'm just the right age."

So I did my thing, and he had a fantastic result with his ACL reconstruction and got back to skiing the black diamonds.

We've really changed our mind-set about how we live, and, as a result, how we should be treated medically and surgically for a variety of conditions. I suppose that's part of the Boomer legacy, but it applies to anyone who strives to be active. I think we (doctors and non-doctors) are reinventing what age really is. We want to keep our bodies going and use technology to have smaller surgeries and heal faster and better.

And, quite frankly, I don't mind treating older folks, and what we now call the mature athlete. They're not anxious, not looking at their watches. They're not sitting there with their parents and saying the next season starts in May, so just fix it. Instead, they want to know everything, and they want to follow every prescription to the letter—the kind of patients any doctor would love to have.

The old, drawn-out procedure came with a higher risk of infection and caused more inflammation, swelling, stiffness, weakness, and scar tissue than the way we do things now. The slew of bad things that could happen way back when is a thing of the past, and, instead of 3 or 4 days in a hospital, a cast for 2 months, and a year of rehab therapy before you could even think about normal activity, you can expect an overnight stay at most, no post-op cast or brace in most instances, and back to feeling pretty normal in a couple of weeks or so. (If "normal" for you is high-level recreation, be advised that it takes 6 to 9 months in most cases for a graft to become strong enough to withstand higher-level rehab drills and competitive running/cutting sports.)

With today's arthroscopy, you wind up feeling good much sooner in terms of getting around, back to the gym, and back to work, but you still have to wait months to really test-drive your newly restrung knee. This becomes a real challenge, especially with younger patients, who think that as soon as the swelling is down and the limp is gone, they are ready for prime time—one of the main reasons for re-tears and stretched-out grafts. ACL surgery is a major commitment to follow the staged rehabilitation necessary for optimal recovery. It's not enough to be 100 percent back; you need to be better than you were before you tore your ACL if you want to avoid a graft tear and revision surgery, which is much more complicated and has a much higher failure rate. Bottom line? Your first shot is your best shot for long-term success.

JOINT DISCUSSION

I usually do ACL reconstructions on Fridays and have my patients come back to the office on Monday just for a quick check. Some of them are already walking without crutches, and you wouldn't know they had had anything done.

I often find myself slowing my patients down. We minimized the surgery so much that patients, especially kids, feel so good after a month or 6 weeks that they're raring to go all-out. We surgeons know better; we have been able to drastically reduce the invasiveness of the procedure, have sped up the initial recovery period, and improved the overall comfort level of the experience, but we haven't been able to speed up the time it takes for the graft to fully incorporate into the body. It will attach properly if you treat it right and do the right kind of therapy, but it continues to remodel and grow for months, and it won't be at full strength until a year-and-a-half later.

KNEEPAD

It takes 18 months in most cases for an ACL graft to not only become part of your body, but, more important, to remodel and achieve its full strength.

We need to do better with ACL surgery. The ACL re-tear rate of 15 percent is too high for my liking, and maybe a full year of rehab is the way to go. And once you start talking about revision surgeries, the failure rate could be as high as 25 percent. The body just doesn't have the same healing response, the same level of scar tissue formation, the second (or sixth, like Picabo Street) time around.

Until the healing process is sped up (that's where new technology comes in), plan on having a long recovery from ACL reconstruction if you want the best possible results. But no matter how accelerated the healing is, you still have to retrain your body, work on your particular risk factors, and manage the things you can't change. For example, if you're loose-jointed, the graft will take on that characteristic as it becomes part of your body and be a little looser than it was when it was put in. It's similar to bypass surgery patients who experience coronary artery disease in their new arteries within a few years because they have a genetic predisposition toward high cholesterol and other cardiovascular disease causes, or because they went right back to the lifestyle that clogged their own arteries in the first place.

A word about partial, or Grade 2, ACL injuries. They are not very common, and most, unfortunately, will go on to become complete tears. I try to manage adults more conservatively with exercise and bracing. Teenagers, on the other hand, are usually best managed with full ACL reconstruction, since they are at such high risk to go on to a complete tear. In select cases, in both adults and younger patients, I have had success tightening or re-tensioning the stretched ACL with a simple arthroscopic outpatient procedure using thermal energy. An arthroscopic probe, or thermal wand, is used to perform this "thermal shrinkage." Research studies have suggested that this doesn't usually work, but I have found just the opposite if patients are selected appropriately. Another newer technique, pioneered by Dr. Richard Steadman, involves a "microfracture" of the damaged ligament and surrounding bone which then creates a "healing response" and a tighter ligament. Clearly,

JOINT DISCUSSION

Not everyone who has a torn ACL has surgery to correct it. For example, my wife had an ACL tear many years ago, but she never had it fixed because her sister (we now know that this injury does run in families) tore her ACL and had the old-fashioned, big open surgery with a long recovery the way we used to do it when I was a resident. Those folks who did recover and had a knee that was more stable after the procedure didn't always fully recover from the surgery itself and the effects of wearing a cast for a long time, which was at least 4 to 6 weeks. The leg would be stiff and weak, and the handful of people who did make it all the way back had to go through an awful lot of dedicated work for a year or more to get there.

Most patients who had the old-style knee operation ended up with a knee that did not work very well and was very susceptible to arthritis. My wife saw her sister go through all of this and knows that she still has a lot of trouble with her knee (her graft actually failed and stretched out over time). She chose not to have reconstructive surgery, and she manages (there's that word again) fine, running 10 miles a couple times a week and going to the gym on schedule. Straight-line activities are usually not a problem in an ACL-deficient knee. Cutting, twisting, and jumping sports and activities are another thing altogether for most individuals with ACL instability.

What I worry about is we still have young kids who are just learning to ski. I've decided that prudent management of my own balky knee precludes the vigorous schussing required to keep an eye on them; my wife, however, will slap a brace on her knee and go out to the slopes with them, tempting fate every time.

more research is needed in both of these techniques, but they are very promising for those with partial tears of their ACL.

Surgical treatment of a **posterior cruciate ligament** sprain is more controversial. Unlike treatment of an ACL tear, there is little agreement about the best way to proceed. I treat most PCL tears conservatively mostly with ice, elevation, braces, and crutches. Once symptoms have settled, physical therapy

Most people who have a PCL tear can get by with conservative treatment. Even football players can play at a high level using a brace and physical therapy because backward laxity can be tolerated much better than forward laxity (as seen in ACL tears) can. However, if you're having exceptional trouble, the PCL can be repaired with a procedure similar to ACL reconstruction.

improves knee motion and strength, and most individuals get back to full unrestricted activity with little or no symptoms. Sometimes a brace is needed for sports.

Surgical reconstruction is usually only recommended for Grade 3 PCL tears in very select patients who are having significant problems despite conservative treatment.

Collateral Ligament Sprains

Partial tears are more common in collateral ligaments than in cruciate ligaments, and they usually respond well to conservative treatment, such as nursing them along with crutches, a brace, and physical therapy for a couple of weeks. The more significant tears need to be protected longer from further trauma so the degree of injury is not worsened.

Today, a medial collateral ligament injury rarely requires surgery. It is interesting to note that when I was in training, we were taught to surgically fix the MCL and usually ignore the ACL. We've completely switched that to where we repair the ACL and just brace and protect the MCL until it heals on its own. An exception is when someone gets hit so hard on the knee, as can happen on a playing field or in a motorcycle accident, that we don't have any choice other than multiple repairs.

Stress Fractures

Other than rest, taking calcium and vitamin D supplements (if intake is usually low, as is the case with many patients, especially females), minimizing the load on an affected bone, and the passage of time, the only other options that are sometimes used for stress fractures are casts and/or ultrasound therapy. While the mechanism by which ultrasound helps fractures to heal is not known, because bones grow in response to physical stress, the healing may be the result of the intense mechanical pressure that its pulsing waves deliver. The Sonic Accelerated Fracture Healing System from Exogen Systems is a handheld, battery-operated device that delivers pulses directly through the skin or, if necessary, through a small hole in a cast. Professional athletes and dancers, for whom every day counts, can now use this device at home to treat stress fractures. (There are other bone stimulators available that have similar effectiveness in helping stubborn fractures to heal.)

Knock-Knees or Bowlegged Knees

If a structural misalignment is causing chronic pain because of wear on one side of the knee or the other, we can do a procedure called an osteotomy: After precise calculations, a small wedge of bone is removed from the top of the tibia or the bottom of the femur to bring the frame back into normal alignment.

Partial or Total Knee Degeneration

If medications and other treatments, along with changing your activity level and using walking supports, are no longer helpful, you and your surgeon will discuss a partial (uni-compartment) or total knee arthroplasty procedure that replaces worn-out parts. As always, my first objective is to keep patients on their own knee parts for as long as possible,

JOINT DISCUSSION

If I can buy 10 or so years for a patient by doing a cartilage regeneration procedure, or by recommending a partial, uni-compartmental knee replacement, I've done that patient a favor because I've built an acceptable bridge to a total knee replacement down the road (if there is no other choice then). Patients often ask me why I don't just put a whole new knee in now, and replace that one when it wears out, like changing parts at the auto dealership. Sure, that can be done, but knee replacements do not come with a lifetime warranty, and each revision gets harder and harder on the patient, on the surgeon, and on the recovery. In addition, more complications are possible with each revision, so if I can keep a patient on his or her own knee as long as possible, with a less-invasive surgery, my patient is better off.

so I use the most conservative treatment at first whenever that is appropriate.

The design of uni-compartmental replacement parts has improved over the years, as has the sophistication of the instruments used to implant them. There's a relatively new technique for those who have kneecap arthritis (patellofemoral arthritis) and the rest of the joint is fine, whereby we replace the cushion behind the kneecap area only and spare the remainder of the joint.

A uni-compartmental replacement procedure requires a smaller incision, and it heals much faster than a total replacement. It feels more normal than a total knee replacement, and you can return to normal activities much sooner, but less than 10 percent of those who have arthritic knees are good candidates for this procedure.

Total knee replacements were first done in 1968, and there are almost 600,000 of these procedures performed every year. (Again, because of our aging Boomer population and the almost universal desire today to remain as active as possible, that number is expected to increase exponentially over the coming decades, off the charts, really, to the point where I doubt there will be enough orthopedic surgeons to handle the volume.) Most patients who undergo this procedure are 60 to 80 years old, but orthopedic surgeons evaluate patients on an individual basis. We are seeing more and more osteoarthritis and worn-out knees in younger and younger patients, and that presents a major therapeutic challenge. This is

KNEEPAD

When It May Be Time for a New Hinge

- An x-ray shows significant arthritis, or it's seen at the time of arthroscopy

- Severe pain limits everyday activities such as walking, climbing stairs, and getting in and out of chairs

- Moderate or severe knee pain while resting, either day or night

- Chronic inflammation and swelling that does not improve with medications

- Failure to obtain pain relief from Tylenol, NSAIDs, joint supplements, and physical therapy

- Failure to obtain relief from cortisone injections, viscosupplementation, and other interventions

- Progressive arthritis-related knee stiffness: inability to bend and/or straighten your knee

- Knee deformity

- A painful arthritic knee that is ruling your life and causing you to change your everyday plans fueled by the beat-up Baby Boomer population, as well as by the obesity epidemic.

Total knee replacements have been performed successfully at all ages, from the young teenager with juvenile arthritis to the elderly patient with degenerative arthritis. Recommendations for surgery are based on a patient's pain and disability, not strictly age, but the younger you are when you first get one, the more likely you are to require future revision surgery, which is not a picnic.

Many different types of designs and materials are currently used in total knee replacement surgery that has three components: the femoral component (made of a highly polished strong metal), the tibial component (made of a durable plastic often held in a metal tray), and the patellar component (also plastic). The procedure usually takes only 1 to 2 hours to go "from skin to skin," but anesthesia has to be administered and a hospital stay for recovery and rehab is required.

A recent advance for total knee replacement is the use of a minimally invasive surgical (MIS) approach. This technique, still in its relative infancy, is more challenging than standard total knee replacement, but more and more joint replacement surgeons are developing the skills to provide this less-invasive approach to their patients. MIS incisions are approximately half the size of those used in a standard approach, and fewer of the important deeper structures, like the quadriceps muscle, are violated. Advantages such as a quicker rehabilitation, less pain, and a shorter hospitalization result. This option is appropriate for non-obese patients who do not have a significant deformity and who have reasonable motion in the joint prior to surgery.

Another newer option for women is the "gender knee" that was designed to provide a

KNEEPAD

Among all types of surgical procedures done, knee replacement enjoys one of the highest success rates and patient satisfaction scores. Also, the complication rate following total knee replacement is low. Blood clots in the leg veins are the most common complication. Serious complications, such as a knee joint infection, occur in fewer than 2 percent of patients. Major medical complications such as heart attack or stroke occur even less frequently. (Chronic illnesses and obesity may increase the potential for complications.)

better fit for females. Theoretically, this makes sense as there are some gender differences in the shape and dimensions around the knee area. Scientific studies, however, have yet to prove better results, and many joint replacement specialists think this may be more marketing than science. Time will tell. One thing for certain is that it is better to have a great surgeon rather than any one specific type of implant, gender, uni, MIS, or whatever is coming next to an O.R. near you.

To restore normal movement in your knee and leg, your surgeon may have you use the CPM machine (mentioned previously) that slowly moves your knee while you are in bed. It decreases leg swelling by elevating your leg, and it actually helps with pain control. CPM may help you regain motion, something that can be very difficult in the first few weeks after knee replacement, but the machine never takes the place of the exercises that you need to do to regain knee mobility. Also, foot and ankle movement is encouraged immediately after surgery to increase bloodflow in your leg muscles and help prevent leg swelling and blood clots. Your recovery protocol should also include medication to prevent these potentially fatal blood clots (also known as a deep vein thrombosis or DVT).

More than 90 percent of individuals who undergo total knee replacement experience a dramatic reduction of knee pain and a significant improvement in their ability to perform common activities of daily living. You get your life back! Total knee replacement, however, will not make you a super-athlete,

KNEEPAD

Questions to Ask Your Knee-Replacement Surgeon

- How many knee replacements do you perform per year?

- Do you do the majority of the case yourself?

- If you use a team of professionals, what do you do and what do they do?

- How accessible are you post-procedure (in the hospital and after I get home)?

- What is your complication rate?

- What are your protocols for preventing infection and blood clots?

- Will I need to go to a rehab facility after I leave the hospital?

- Are there any alternatives to knee replacement for me?

and you must have reasonable expectations as to what you can and can't do. Following surgery, you will be advised to avoid kneeling as well as some types of activity, including jogging and high-impact sports, for the rest of your life, but you will be able to exercise and remain fit, or get back into shape if you had let things slip.

One final comment about total knee arthroplasty: Picking your surgeon is critical. You should work only with someone who does at least 100 procedures every year, has a great reputation, and does most of the procedure himself or herself. Be wary of anyone who is too marketing-oriented or has an assembly line going. (I could do a lot more volume and make more dough, but that isn't my style. I spend more time with people, and I wouldn't be happy if I didn't serve my patients that way. I often ask patients, "Do you want fast food, or cooked-to-order?" Most of them understand the connection to good patient care and communication.)

PAST, PRESENT, AND FUTURE

The scope is indeed a wonderful tool and the artificial knee is a technological miracle, but to me, we've failed when we reach that endgame because we weren't able to preserve Mother Nature's marvelous original equipment.

KNEEPAD

Joint Class

Many hospitals offer "joint classes" for individuals scheduled for or contemplating joint replacement surgery. I think they are wonderful. Patients meet with nurses, physical therapists, and many other members of the hospital team that will be taking care of them pre- and post-operatively. You learn so much more than any physician can offer during busy office sessions. You also get multiple perspectives (often more accurate than the picture the surgeon paints), and you can ask all the questions you desire. I recommend them wholeheartedly and sincerely believe they should be mandatory.

I am reminded of a patient who came to my office for a knee arthroscopy, not a knee replacement. He was a very famous, hair-down-to-his-waist hippie and radio rock-and-roll DJ. He looked over at a sign in the waiting room advertising the "joint classes" at our local hospital, and his eyebrows raised in delight. "That's cool," he said. "Do they show you how to roll them and all?" I don't think he was kidding.

I have said again and again that a surgeon's first goal should be prevention. We are spending more than one trillion dollars on health care in the United States, and only about 2 percent of that goes to avoiding treatment of disease and surgical and other invasive procedures. The rest is spent on patchwork after things go wrong. We will never solve out-of-control costs until our focus shifts from being Dr. Fix-Its to prevention experts. New treatments are fantastic, even magical, but they're expensive and evermore so. It might be biting the hand that feeds me, but much better value for our dollars comes from investing in approaches that keep people out of my office.

I recovered from a traumatic knee injury in my youth, and a few decades went by before any other symptoms cropped up, because I lived healthy and stayed active. If I had been a couch potato, I don't know that I would have ever gotten back to being able to play sports at a high level back then, or able to recreate like I do now. We've got great technology today, and better stuff is coming tomorrow, but nothing is better than preventing problems in the first place.

How can you do that? Take the next three steps.

"KNOODLE" THIS

Pain should not be the only warning light you have that something is amiss. Although it is usually temporary, and not necessarily an indication that something is terribly wrong, you don't have to wait until pain shows up to take action on a health issue.

Part of every *FrameWork* edition is a self-check test that identifies weak links in the chain of wellness, and in some cases even exposes a potential time bomb. The short questionnaire that follows is designed to pick up muscle imbalances, weakness, or atrophy; deficits in balance or proprioception (fine-tune coordination, for anyone who needs a reminder); loss of range of motion; and lifestyle issues that merit attention. All of these are issues that can really mess up your frame if left unchecked; these "weak links" or vulnerabilities often fly under the radar, waiting for the opportunity to rear their heads.

The test is vital to everything that follows, because you can't very well work with what you have unless you know where you are to begin with. In less than 30 minutes, you'll have a snapshot of how your knees fare now and how you will be able to make them better. You'll breeze through the majority of questions in about 5 minutes, and the rest of the time will be spent on "getting physical"—completing some exercises and maneuvers that assess the critical support structure of your knees.

KNEEPAD

There's an interactive comprehensive self-test for your *entire* frame, with forms you can print out, on my Web site, www.drnick.com.

The scoring system I devised for your test follows the scheme my mechanic uses when he goes over my car. Every aspect gets the once-over and a color rating:

Green means smooth sailing.

Yellow means something needs to be watched and/or worked on.

Red means let's do something *right now* about it.

I've used this color-coded approach for many years with athletes and active individuals in my practice, and I know that it gets to the heart of the matter very quickly. Circle the appropriate color for each question below (and be brutally honest, or you'll only be fooling yourself). If you circle any "red" responses, be sure to discuss them with your doctor and proceed with caution in Step 5 after he or she gives you the green light to do so.

HISTORY

1. Do you have a family history of significant knee problems?

a. No	green
b. Yes	yellow
c. Major knee surgery	red

2. Do you wear out your shoes unevenly, one shoe versus the other?

(Take a pair of well-worn, but not worn out, shoes or sneakers and look from behind at the heel and/or inner arch area. Also look underneath at the wear patterns on the sole, both front and back.)

a. They're the same	green
b. Maybe a slight difference	yellow
c. It's like night and day	red

3. Do you ever limp because of your knee?

a. No	green
b. Rarely after a hard workout	yellow
c. Yes, my rapper name would be Sir Limp-A-Lot	red

4. Does your knee ever "catch" or "lock"?

a. No	green
b. I sometimes get a catching or clicking sensation as I straighten it, but it straightens okay	yellow
c. My knee gets stuck in a bent position, and at times I can't get it straight	red

5. Does your knee ever "give way" or buckle?

a. No	green
b. It sometimes feels like it might give way, but I usually catch myself	yellow
c. My knee goes out more than I do	red

6. Are your joints hypermobile? To find out:

1. Hyperextend (go beyond straight) your elbows

2. Hyperextend (go beyond straight) your knees

3. Try to pull your thumb all the way backward to touch your forearm or pull your fingers all the way back so they are at a right angle or beyond to your hand

a. My joints do not hyperextend	green
b. One or more joints slightly hyperextend	yellow
c. Call me Gumby!	red

7. Are you female? (Sorry, ladies, but women are at higher risk for a variety of knee problems.)

a. No	green
b. Yes	yellow
c. I am a teenage girl who enjoys running/cutting, sudden stop-start sports, and activities like soccer, basketball, field hockey, lacrosse, and skiing	red

8. Have any siblings or immediate family members ever torn their ACL?

a. No	green
b. Yes	red

9. Do you have any stiffness in your knee upon awakening (i.e., until showering or moving around for a while), after sitting still for more than 30 minutes, or for no apparent reason?

a. No	green
b. Only the day after a hard workout	yellow
c. It's a part of my life	red

10. Do your knees creak or make noise going up or down stairs?

a. No	green
b. Yes, but there's no discomfort or pain	yellow
c. Yes, and it does cause discomfort or pain	red

11. Do you have trouble ascending or descending stairs?

a. No	green
b. Only after going up and down multiple times, especially while carrying heavier items	yellow
c. Yes	red

12. Do changes in barometric pressure (especially damp, rainy weather) make your knee(s) ache?

a. No	green
b. Rarely	yellow
c. Friends consult me instead of the weatherman	red

13. Do you find that you change your plans or activities because of a knee problem?

a. No	green
b. Occasionally (no more than a few times a year)	yellow
c. Yes, my knee is beginning to rule my life	red

14. Do you have difficulty falling asleep at night or awaken during the night because of knee discomfort?

a. No	green
b. Rarely, or minor difficulty	yellow
c. It's a struggle as soon as my head hits the pillow	red

15. Have you had to see a doctor or other health-care provider in the past 3 years for a knee problem?

a. No	green
b. One or two visits	yellow
c. I get frequent-flier miles at the orthopedic office	red

16. Have you ever had a knee injury that was severe enough to require crutches and/or keep you out of sports or exercise for an extended period?

a. No	green
b. I was hobbled, but not for long	yellow
c. I was out of action for a month or more	red

17. Have you ever dislocated or subluxed your patella?

a. No	green
b. Yes	red

18. Do you have knee swelling?

a. No	green
b. Rarely, and only if I really push myself	yellow
c. You mean that's not normal?	red

19. Have you lost mobility (range of motion) in either knee? For example, are you unable to fully straighten (extend) and fully bend (flex) them?

a. No	green
b. A little stiff at times, but motion is full	yellow
c. Motion is limited one or both ways	red

20. Have you ever had knee surgery?

a. No	green
b. It looms as a possibility	yellow
c. Yes	red

LIFESTYLE

1. For how many hours at a stretch do you sit at a desk?

a. Less than 2	green
b. 2 to 4	yellow
c. More than 4	red

2. Have you ever smoked?

a. No	green
b. Not in the past 10 years	yellow
c. I'm planning to quit	red

3. Find your spot on the BMI chart on page 70—are you significantly overweight?

a. Good weight (BMI below 25)	green
b. Mild overweight (BMI 25 to 29)	yellow
c. Overweight and/or obese (BMI 30 or over)	red

4. What's your daily consumption of fruits and vegetables?

a. Seven to nine servings and a rainbow of colors	green
b. Maybe a green salad with dinner	yellow
c. Does ketchup qualify as a vegetable?	red

5. How often do you eat oily, cold-water fish, such as salmon or sardines?

a. Once or twice a week	green
b. A couple of times a month	yellow
c. Do Cheddar Goldfish crackers count?	red

6. Do you take a daily multivitamin and also get sufficient vitamin D as well as antioxidants (vitamins A, C, and E via food or supplement)?

a. Never miss a day	green
b. I could be more consistent	yellow
c. Who has the time?	red

7. Do you routinely need to take Advil, Aleve, Motrin, or prescription drugs for knee discomfort?

a. No	green
b. Once or twice a month	yellow
c. I make sure to never run out	red

8. Do you have to take prescription narcotic drugs for knee pain?

a. No	green
b. On rare occasions (i.e., once or twice a year)	yellow
c. Pretty regularly, or almost every day and/or for extended periods of time	red

9. How much water do you take in a day?

a. 8 full glasses	green
b. 4 to 6 glasses, usually	yellow
c. I'm more of a camel—I go extended periods without a sip	red

10. How often do you work out?

a. Three times a week, an hour a day	green
b. Maybe once or twice a week	yellow
c. I've been meaning to join a gym	red

11. What does your workout consist of?

a. Balanced routines including aerobic, strengthening, stretching, and core work	green
b. A little of this and a little of that	yellow
c. Mostly one thing (running, yoga, swimming, weights)	red

12. If you're a runner, how many miles do you log in a week?

a. Less than 25	green
b. 25 to 30	yellow
c. 30+	red

Body Mass Index Table

Body Weight (pounds)

Height (inches)	Normal						Overweight					Obese										Extreme Obesity														
BMI	19	20	21	22	23	24	25	26	27	28	29	30	31	32	33	34	35	36	37	38	39	40	41	42	43	44	45	46	47	48	49	50	51	52	53	54
58	91	96	100	105	110	115	119	124	129	134	138	143	148	153	158	162	167	172	177	181	186	191	196	201	205	210	215	220	224	229	234	239	244	248	253	258
59	94	99	104	109	114	119	124	128	133	138	143	148	153	158	163	168	173	178	183	188	193	198	203	208	212	217	222	227	232	237	242	247	252	257	262	267
60	97	102	107	112	118	123	128	133	138	143	148	153	158	163	168	174	179	184	189	194	199	204	209	215	220	225	230	235	240	245	250	255	261	266	271	276
61	100	106	111	116	122	127	132	137	143	148	153	158	164	169	174	180	185	190	195	201	206	211	217	222	227	232	238	243	248	254	259	264	269	275	280	285
62	104	109	115	120	126	131	136	142	147	153	158	164	169	175	180	186	191	196	202	207	213	218	224	229	235	240	246	251	256	262	267	273	278	284	289	295
63	107	113	118	124	130	135	141	146	152	158	163	169	175	180	186	191	197	203	208	214	220	225	231	237	242	248	254	259	265	270	278	282	287	293	299	304
64	110	116	122	128	134	140	145	151	157	163	169	174	180	186	192	197	204	209	215	221	227	232	238	244	250	256	262	267	273	279	285	291	296	302	308	314
65	114	120	126	132	138	144	150	156	162	168	174	180	186	192	198	204	210	216	222	228	234	240	246	252	258	264	270	276	282	288	294	300	306	312	318	324
66	118	124	130	136	142	148	155	161	167	173	179	186	192	198	204	210	216	223	229	235	241	247	253	260	266	272	278	284	291	297	303	309	315	322	328	334
67	121	127	134	140	146	153	159	166	172	178	185	191	198	204	211	217	223	230	236	242	249	255	261	268	274	280	287	293	299	306	312	319	325	331	338	344
68	125	131	138	144	151	158	164	171	177	184	190	197	203	210	216	223	230	236	243	249	256	262	269	276	282	289	295	302	308	315	322	328	335	341	348	354
69	128	135	142	149	155	162	169	176	182	189	196	203	209	216	223	230	236	243	250	257	263	270	277	284	291	297	304	311	318	324	331	338	345	351	358	365
70	132	139	146	153	160	167	174	181	188	195	202	209	216	222	229	236	243	250	257	264	271	278	285	292	299	306	313	320	327	334	341	348	355	362	369	376
71	136	143	150	157	165	172	179	186	193	200	208	215	222	229	236	243	250	257	265	272	279	286	293	301	308	315	322	329	338	343	351	358	365	372	379	386
72	140	147	154	162	169	177	184	191	199	206	213	221	228	235	242	250	258	265	272	279	287	294	302	309	316	324	331	338	346	353	361	368	375	383	390	397
73	144	151	159	166	174	182	189	197	204	212	219	227	235	242	250	257	265	272	280	288	295	302	310	318	325	333	340	348	355	363	371	378	386	393	401	408
74	148	155	163	171	179	186	194	202	210	218	225	233	241	249	256	264	272	280	287	295	303	311	319	326	334	342	350	358	365	373	381	389	396	404	412	420
75	152	160	168	176	184	192	200	208	216	224	232	240	248	256	264	272	279	287	295	303	311	319	327	335	343	351	359	367	375	383	391	399	407	415	423	431
76	156	164	172	180	189	197	205	213	221	230	238	246	254	263	271	279	287	295	304	312	320	328	336	344	353	361	369	377	385	394	402	410	418	426	435	443

Source: Adapted from *Clinical Guidelines on the Identification, Evaluation, and Treatment of Overweight and Obesity in Adults: The Evidence Report.*

13. Do you run to get in shape, or get in shape to run?

a. I am in shape, or I'll walk, swim, bike (or other low-impact alternatives) till I'm buffed and ready to run	green
b. I'm out of shape and/or overweight, and I'll run a little to burn extra calories	yellow
c. Running is the best and only way to lose those pounds	red

14. For a given sport or activity (bicycling, Rollerblading, skateboarding), do you wear the full protective gear suggested?

a. Yes	green
b. Usually	yellow
c. No	red

15. Do you stop an activity when you feel pain?

a. Always	green
b. Usually	yellow
c. "No pain, no gain" is my mantra	red

16. Do you need to wear a knee brace, sleeve, or support for activities?

a. No	green
b. I need it for tougher activities and sports	yellow
c. No sports for me unless I'm wrapped or braced, and my friends sometimes yell, "Run, Forrest, run!"	red

17. How much sleep do you get each night?

a. 7 to 8 hours	green
b. One hour over or under that span	yellow
c. A lot more (or a lot less)	red

18. Is your sleep restful?

a. I can't wait to face each day	green
b. I often wake up tired, and some afternoons really drag	yellow
c. I check the clock during the night a lot more than I'd like	red

GET PHYSICAL

Caution: These tests may not be easy, but they should be comfortable and not result in any pain. If there is significant discomfort with any of these tests, or if you are unable to perform one or more, *stop* doing those tests and score a "red." Then check with your physician or other health-care professional.

The same rules apply here that apply to any good workout:

■ Warm up before you begin

■ Use slow, controlled movements

■ No bouncing or ballistic movements

■ No forcing beyond comfort

■ No pain

■ Remember: It's not a competition

1. Knee and Leg Alignment

Stand barefoot, facing a mirror, and put your legs together. Look in the mirror. For most of us, our knees will touch slightly, and there may be an inch between our ankles. (A doctor can check this with a standing x-ray of your knee to confirm.) If your knees are touching and your ankles are inches apart, you have a Valgus alignment—you're knock-kneed. If your ankles are together and your knees are apart, you have a Varus alignment—you're bowlegged.

a. Legs line up pretty straight	green
b. Ankles together and 1 inch between knees or knees together and up to 2 inches between ankles	yellow
c. Ankles together and more than 1 inch between knees or knees together and more than 2 inches between ankles	red

2. Kneecap Alignment

Stand facing a mirror, feet together and pointing straight ahead.

Are your kneecaps pointing inward, outward, or straight ahead? Place an imaginary dot in the center of the kneecap to help you visualize the path of the kneecap, then picture water squirting straight out from the dots. Is it shooting forward, parallel in the general direction of your feet and toes, or way off inward with the water streams crossing, or outward away from your body?

a. Straight ahead	green
b. Slightly in or out, but still aiming in the same direction as my feet	yellow
c. Aiming way outward or inward	red

3. The Stork (Basic Balance)

Stand up straight, extend your arms out wide to your sides, then raise one foot off the ground up to the level of the opposite knee (see photo). Rest the arch of your foot on the inner side of your knee, forming the letter "P." Now close your eyes. Repeat with your opposite side. How long can you stay balanced that way?

a. 30 seconds	green
b. 15 to 29 seconds	yellow
c. Less than 15 seconds	red

4. The Horse

With knees splayed out like you are on a very large horse or small hippo, go into a partial squat (knees bent not quite to 90 degrees). Look straight ahead and hold up to 90 seconds. If you are unable to do the "horse," try doing the "wall seat" easier version (see page 123). How was your "ride"?

a. Can hold for 90 seconds then rise easily;
   actually found it a little relaxing — green

b. Struggled some; I could get down fine, but
   getting up was hard, or I could hold for 30 seconds
   but my legs, they were a-shakin'! — yellow

c. You won't see me at the Kentucky Derby, 'cause
   I can't ride that horse hardly at all — red

5. Hop Test

Hop on each foot, 20 times right and 20 times left. (**Note:** You should have equal spring with fairly quiet landings. A weak leg would go "thud" or your form will begin to deteriorate.)

a. You can go 20 times without weakening — green

b. After 10, your pace becomes a problem or it's uncomfortable — yellow

c. No can do, or there's a difference between right and left sides — red

6. Quadriceps Test

Wearing shorts, sit on the floor with your legs extended forward and your muscles relaxed. Use a pen to make a mark on the front of your thigh, 4 inches above the upper or proximal edge of your kneecap. Mark the exact same spot on the other leg, measuring again from the top of the kneecap. Next, measure the circumference of each thigh at that exact level using a tape measure or string. As you are measuring, gently straighten the leg while it remains on the ground, tightening the thigh muscle. While measuring, do not pull the tape or string tightly to compress the thigh muscle; just pull it gently to get the exact circumference. Compare the measurements of your thighs.

a. Equal	green
b. Less than ½-inch difference	yellow
c. ½-inch or more difference	red

7. Calf Test

Sit in a chair and cross your legs. Measure the circumference of your calf at its largest area while relaxed. Repeat for the opposite side. Compare measurements. (**Note:** When your knee is bad, the entire leg may be weaker, or the calf muscle on the involved side may actually be bigger as your body compensates for the weak knee.)

a. Equal	green
b. Less than ¼-inch difference	yellow
c. ¼-inch or more difference	red

8. Single-Leg Calf Raise

Stand on one foot with your other toes on the first step of a stairway or on a large, stable book. Let your heel drop down so that the heel is lower than the toes by approximately 1 inch at the start of each repetition. Do not "spring" up; rather, do slow, controlled lifts, both up and down. How many calf raises (going as high as possible) can you do with your left leg, then with your right leg?

a. 20 or more	green
b. 10 to 19	yellow
c. Fewer than 10	red

9. Hamstring Tightness Test

Sit on the floor with your feet flat against a wall, with your feet pointing upward and your ankles at a 90-degree angle. Sit tall (as if a string were pulling the top of your head toward the ceiling) and reach forward (like a walking zombie), with your index fingers touching side by side. While staying tall and keeping your chest high, slowly lean forward, keeping your knees straight, and try to touch the wall (at the level of your eyes, i.e., don't reach down toward your toes but stay tall with good sitting posture). How did you do?

a. Can place both palms on the wall	green
b. Can reach the wall only with my fingertips	yellow
c. Can't reach the wall	red

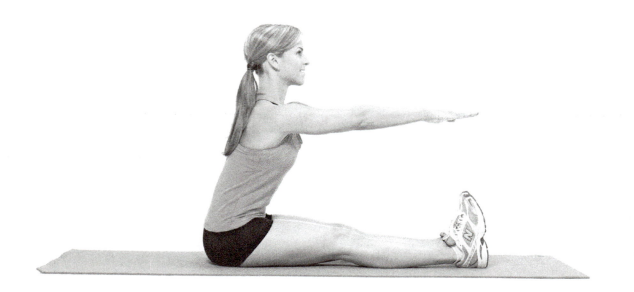

10. Alternate Hamstring Tightness Test

If you have really long arms (and you know who you are), then you might be able to reach the wall even if you have tight hamstrings. Double-check with this alternative test.

Lie on your back with your legs out straight. Gently flex the hip of one leg, bringing the knee up toward you until the hip is at 90 degrees with your knee still bent. Keeping the hip at 90 degrees (don't let it drop back down), slowly straighten your knee fully until the leg is out straight and the heel is pointing toward the ceiling. (This test is easier to visualize if you lie sideways to a mirror so you can watch your positioning.) Repeat with your opposite side. How did you do?

a. Leg goes up beyond "L" position with no strain	green
b. Knee gets almost fully straight but feels tight	yellow
c. Knee is too tight to fully straighten leg	red

11. Quadriceps Tightness Test

Lie on your stomach with your legs extended, knees close together. Keep your knees touching; don't let them drift apart. Bend your left leg at the knee (or have a friend gently help), bringing your left foot up toward your buttock. Your left heel should be able to touch your buttock while you remain absolutely flat against the floor. Repeat with your opposite side. If your quadriceps are too tight, either your heel won't reach your buttock, or you'll have to tilt your pelvis or buttocks area off the floor to accommodate. How did you do?

a. Heel reaches buttock easily	green
b. Can do, but feeling of tightness in front of thigh	yellow
c. Heel can't reach buttock, or pelvis tilts (lifts up)	red

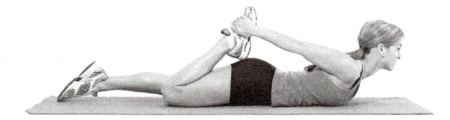

12. Iliotibial Band Test

Lie on your left side with your legs straight. Flex your right knee and grab your right foot, bringing your right heel toward your butt. Keeping the rest of your body straight (i.e., your spine, pelvis, and left leg), pull your right foot, letting your right knee go back 2 to 3

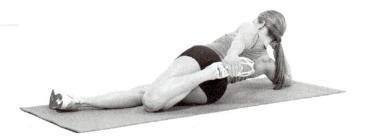

inches, and then allow your right knee to drop back and down behind your left knee, touching the floor. Repeat with your opposite side. What does your knee do?

a. Knee easily drops back and down to the floor	green
b. Knee drops down but is 2 to 3 inches from the floor	yellow
c. Knee hangs up and does not drop much	red

13. Hip Tightness Test

Lie on a stable tabletop (or off the end of the bed) with your knees and lower legs hanging over the end. Bring both of your knees up until they are clutched to your chest in a "cannonball" position. Now, while one leg remains snug in that position, slowly lower the other. You should be able to place this other knee back fully flat on the table with your leg once again dangling over the side without your other hip coming down or your pelvis rocking forward. If it "hangs up," the front of your hip is too tight. Repeat with the alternate leg. How does it go?

a. Legs go back down fully, easily	green
b. Legs go back down fully, but feel tight in front	yellow
c. Leg or legs do not go down fully	red

14. Core Strength and Endurance (Quadruped)

While kneeling on the floor, place your forearms flat on the floor as if you were going to do a modified pushup. Next, assume the "plank" position, with your body straight and your full weight supported on both forearms and toes (second photo). Your body should be straight as a board with your pelvis tucked inward, and your abdominal and buttock muscles tight. Try holding that position with your weight on your forearms and toes for 60 seconds.

Next, lift your right arm off the floor for 15 seconds, supporting your full weight on your left arm and both feet (third photo). Repeat, lifting your left arm. With both forearms on the floor, raise your right leg, hold for 15 seconds, and then repeat, lifting your left leg.

Next, try to elevate your right arm and left leg simultaneously (fourth photo) and hold for 15 seconds, then return them to the floor and repeat with your left arm and right leg raised. Return to the plank position and hold for 30 seconds. How did it go?

a. Able to do all positions for the required time	green
b. Able to do all positions for half of the required time	yellow
c. Unable to hold all or any positions other than briefly	red

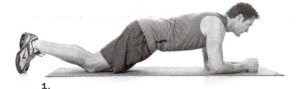

1.

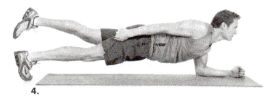

2.

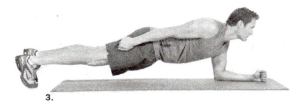

3.

4.

15. Side Plank Test

Start on the floor lying on your left side, propping yourself up on your left forearm with your left elbow in line with your left shoulder, and your left outer thigh and leg on the floor with your feet lying stacked on one another. Your right arm should rest relaxed along your right side with your palm on your right hip. Press your hips toward the ceiling and lift your body off the floor so as to form a straight line, while balancing on your forearm and the side of your foot. Hold this position while contracting your abdominals to stabilize your torso. Breathe comfortably and don't hold your breath. Try to simultaneously tighten your abs and gluteal (butt) muscles, but keep your shoulders relaxed. Time yourself as you hold this position as long as you can comfortably without sagging or squirming. Now try this on the opposite side. How long could you hold?

a. 3 minutes	green
b. less than 3 minutes	yellow
c. less than 30 seconds or can't do	red

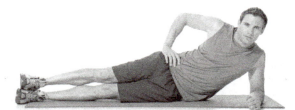

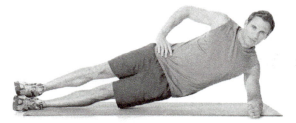

16. Single-Leg Squat Test

Face a mirror and flex your left knee so that you're balancing on your right leg. Next, slowly lower yourself down so that you are squatting halfway down on the right leg and your right thigh is almost parallel to the ground. Repeat on your opposite side. How did you do on each side?

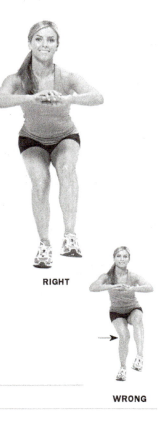

RIGHT

WRONG

a. Able to go down slowly in a controlled fashion,
   and my knee remains directly over my foot   green

b. Able to do it with mild difficulty, and/or my
   knee began to buckle inward a little   yellow

c. My knee buckles well inward, and/or I am unable to do this
   because of pain or weakness   red

17. Jump Test

Caution: You probably should hold off on this test if any of the following are true:

· You're not athletic and not used to jumping.

· You don't do sports and don't plan to.

· Your knee is painful or swollen and/or has instability issues.

· You have knee weakness and/or you had a recent injury or surgery.

· You have balance or fall issues.

In these instances, your doctor or physical therapist can assess these important parameters and determine when the time is right for you to try this.

Research has shown that certain individuals (especially but not only females) are prone to serious knee injuries like ACL tears because of a deficiency in their landing gear. From a biomechanical efficiency standpoint, they don't land properly. Instead of a solid square landing with the knees bent and directly over the feet, those prone to knee injury will land with the knees straight (and/or hyperextended) or they will land flexed, but the knees will buckle inward (toward each other) ever so slightly. There are programs designed to improve the landing gear (see the KneePad on page 9) and lower the incidence of ACL tears and other knee injuries. You can do the jump test in front of a mirror, and it is even better if someone films you doing it. You can even try it a few times in a row to see if you fatigue easily or your form begins to suffer. Also, before trying this on a higher box, platform, or step, you may want to try it on level ground or a small step.

Stand on a solid box or platform approximately 12 inches high (the bottom two steps of a staircase can also work as well as the stackable steps found in aerobic studios). Jump off and land simultaneously onto both feet (pointing forward and parallel). As you get better at this test, you can increase the height of the step or platform and also try jumping higher.

My landing was:

a. Solid, like a cat, knees bent and remaining perfectly over my feet	green
b. Pretty solid, knees bent and over my feet, but I felt a little shaky and could not "stick" the landing, especially if I did it over and over	yellow
c. Give me a parachute—I tend to land with my knee straight and/or they buckle inward every time	red

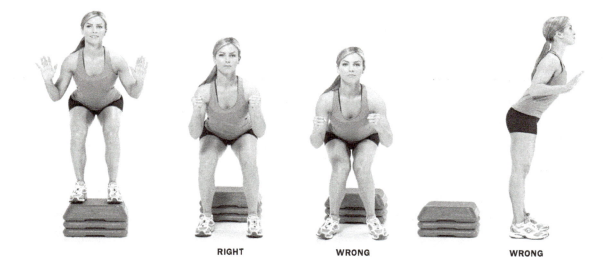

RIGHT   WRONG   WRONG

TOTALS:

green: _____

yellow: _____

red: _____

ASSESSMENT

The above self-evaluation is not so much about a particular "score"; it's about identifying and focusing on critical areas that need your attention so you can lead a more active life. It's less about whether you have passed or failed and more about raising your awareness about the many things that contribute to having a healthy frame.

The more reds you have, the more serious risk you have related to your knees. If you didn't circle any reds but you have a passel of yellows, you're at high risk of slipping into one or more red classifications in the not-too-distant future. If you had just a couple of yellows and the rest were green, you're in good shape and it won't take much to get into top shape. If you circled nothing but green, give yourself a pat on the back (it shouldn't be hard for you to do that, given the tip-top shape you're in), and you should count on doing a more advanced knee routine in Step 5 right from the get-go.

What's most important to take away from this "exercise" is that regardless of what shape you're in, it can be better. Any frame can be made stronger and fine-tune coordination can be made sharper. Any weak links you have can be modified or at least managed better, albeit some more easily than others. (You can monitor your progress by repeating this self-test once or twice a year, or more often if needed, and paying special attention to those questions you answered with a yellow or red.) Take the next two steps and you will make yourself far less vulnerable down the road, and able to rely on the hinges you were born with a whole lot longer.

"Kneed" to Know

You've had a primer on the knee and its woes, and you know a lot more about your weak links. Before you embark on the targeted exercises in the next step that will keep your hinges well oiled, we've got to address the foundation that must support any program. Exercise is a fantastic prescription for health, but there's more to it than exercise alone if you want to achieve optimal musculoskeletal health and a durable frame. Otherwise you might even end up doing more harm than good for yourself.

Anyone who is already familiar with the FrameWork philosophy knows what that entails: a healthy lifestyle, balanced training, core fitness, proper rest and recovery, and a sound mind. A weekly golf or tennis date, or regular visits to the local gym, won't extend your frame's warranty the way this comprehensive approach does.

Medicine advances every day, but there are some things that will never change. If you want to be *active for life,* you've got to address all of the aspects that impact well-being. Even if much of what we cover in this step is familiar to you, it never hurts to revisit the absolutes of frame health. At the top of that list is the subject of widespread public service messages.

SMOKE GETS IN YOUR BONES

Doctors and health officials won't stop beating the anti-smoking drum until the nastiest of habits is a thing of the past for everyone. It bears repeating here that blood vessel constriction caused by smoke inhalation has been linked to poor bone healing and a variety of other negative musculoskeletal consequences, and that many orthopedic surgeons now say they won't operate on someone unless he or she quits.

Smokers have poor bone healing because bones have to rely on micro-circulation, a network of tiny capillaries that is constricted by smoke. Smoking slows or prevents bone healing (what we doctors refer to as delayed unions or non-unions), and smokers have a higher incidence of rotator cuff injuries, degenerative disks, and other frame problems. Even passive smoke exposure could instantly shut down the microvascular networ k of blood vessels. So quit *now,* and shun all who partake. You'll be doing yourself, and them, a favor.

HEAVY BREATHING

Any program to improve health must include moderate aerobic exercise for 30 minutes at least three times per week, and your knee program is no exception. In general, your heart can't tell the difference between different aerobic activities (they all help improve cardiac health and function), but your frame can, as it will certainly have its preferences depending on what ails you. Running is great, but it delivers a pounding to your hinges, so unless you're a die-hard runner with healthy knees, there are other options to get your heart pumping and blood moving that are a lot easier on them (especially if you are one of the many with osteoarthritis brewing in your knee or knees).

Walking

Wear comfortable shoes with good support and cushion and start at a slow pace for 5 minutes to warm up. Increase to a medium pace for 10 minutes, and gradually build up to 30 minutes by adding a few minutes each day. Cool down with 5 minutes at a slow pace. After a few weeks, increase intensity by increasing the pace. (If it's difficult to talk while you walk, you may be overextending yourself—dial it back a notch.)

Water Workouts

If you have access to a pool, swimming, walking, or jogging in the water as well as water aerobic routines are terrific low-impact exercise options, especially for those who are overweight or have knee woes. For a more intense workout, add paddles or other forms of resistance to your upper and lower body.

Stationary Bike

Your seat should be high enough so that your knees are almost but not fully locked out when the pedal is at its lowest. (A recumbent bike is used in a reclining position that is sometimes easier on the knees.) Cycling remains one of the best activities for the knee.

It is a cornerstone of knee rehabilitation because, from an exercise specificity standpoint, it targets the ever important quadriceps muscle better than any other aerobic-type exercise, building both strength and endurance. Think about it: Which athletes have the biggest and strongest thighs? Cyclists do, more so than distance runners. This exercise specificity concept also brings to mind so many patients, whose knees I've operated on, who think that they will regain strength in their quads just because they stand or walk all day long. Not so—one must work the thigh to build the thigh. No way around it.

Elliptical Trainer

This machine is a cross between a stationary bike and a stair-climber. It's a lower-impact activity for the knees than walking, and when the arms are also used (i.e., not just resting on the handles), it provides a higher-intensity cardio workout as it works all of the frame's primary muscle groups. Some individuals with knee problems do better if they cheat a little and hold on to the arm handles.

Intervals and Other Options

Another terrific training option involves the use of interval training. Intervals can be done with any aerobic activity and are accomplished by turning up the intensity for short bursts of time. For example, if you are on a stationary bike, you can increase the resistance for a 30- to 60-second "interval" so you feel like you are climbing a steep hill. Your thighs will scream and burn, but you will rev your metabolism, build quad strength and endurance, and improve your aerobic and anaerobic capacity. Same if you are jogging; add a short sprint. Intervals are a great addition to any aerobic activity. They provide a great training stimulus, are good for your heart and health, and help break up the monotony. They are also effective in getting you off a training plateau that might occur.

If the activities above aren't your cup of tea, take a bicycle to and from work or local stores, or just take it for a long ride around your neighborhood. If you are lucky enough to have healthy knees without arthritis, by all means enjoy jogging! It is hard to find an easier activity than running, but remember, although running does not cause arthritis, it can cause it to worsen or progress if you already have it. So be smart and choose whatever works for you to get your heart pumping without causing harm to any part of your frame. You'll not only get that blood moving, you'll keep your weight down, and that lightens the load on your knees. As an added bonus, through a release of endorphins and systemic hormones, aerobic activity lowers stress, anxiety, and pain levels.

BALANCED TRAINING

"Mirror muscles" might look terrific, but they're not as beautiful as they could be if lesser muscles and the cardiovascular system aren't given a regular workout. In fact, mirror muscles might actually work against you if they are overdeveloped, because they could cause weaker neglected areas to "pop" more than they would if all soft tissues were properly balanced.

Running and other strenuous aerobic activities can also create imbalances. For example, a lot of runners only like to run and will typically have great hearts and very strong calves, but they usually have extremely tight hamstrings, a tight lower back, and relatively weak abdominals, so they're set up for back, hip, and knee problems. Their frame is out of balance because of the disparities created by the repetitive act of running.

If you're a gym rat or a runner, that's great—I'd be the last one to stop anyone from working out. For comprehensive frame health, however, you've got to do some cross-training that includes targeted stretching,

core exercises, and strengthening of all muscle groups to stay out of trouble with any frame part.

"ACTIVE" R & R

Fierce dedication to exercise is laudable, but proper recovery from exercise is a step that is often overlooked by many health-minded individuals. And if you're one of those who think that just alternating workout activities—aerobic training one day, anaerobic the next—is adequate for recovery, you've got another thing coming because your entire body needs to be shut down at times.

Overall stress accumulates in your body, and you aren't aware of that as you go on. Exercises might be directed at one area, but there is a cumulative toll on your system that can cause an overall crash or overuse injury. Overtraining syndrome and overuse injuries are preventable if you give your body the rest that it needs after life-giving, but strenuous, exercise.

Rest must occur both locally (i.e., certain muscles worked) and systemically (from an overall metabolic standpoint). Exercise is a powerful stimulus that creates spectacular changes in your body and frame, but those positive changes occur during the rest and recovery period, which is a critical time for making gains. Come back too soon and apply another stimulus before adequate recovery occurs, and you're asking for a breakdown. It's a lot like cell phones and PDAs—they've transformed how we live and how we communicate, but if you don't routinely recharge their batteries, they're useless. This applies to you, too. Take time, and measures, to recharge.

This doesn't mean you should plop into a recliner and put your feet up. There are better ways to recover from exercise:

- Casual walking
- Stretching
- Yoga
- Meditation

In other words, you can still "do" something (that's why we call it "active" R & R) to gain the benefit of doing nothing. And sometimes, it's even okay to plop on that recliner.

Your nutritional choices (covered in depth in the next section) are also very important in terms of recovery, especially after a hard workout or a few hours of your favorite sport. Muscle recovery is aided by taking in food, drink, or a supplement that contains the right mix of proteins and carbs within 30 minutes of stopping the activity. Interestingly, low-fat chocolate milk has been shown

to be the perfect blend to aid and optimize recovery immediately after a hard workout. (You should also refuel your muscles later that day with a quality high-carb meal.)

The importance of hydration cannot be overstated. It plays a critical role in helping your frame bounce back from the natural wear and tear that exercise causes. Water intake all day long and before, during, and after exercise is a must because it oils your body's repair mechanisms and "juices" that synovial fluid in your knees.

Last, but not least, proper sleep is critical for recovery. Studies show that those who sleep less than 6 hours, or more than 9, have impaired mental function, are more susceptible to disease, and have higher mortality rates. Prolonged periods of disturbed sleep require the attention of a physician. If you are not among the 40 million of those who have a chronic sleep disorder, but you have an

KNEEPAD

Lao Tsu on Overexertion

(from the *Tao Te Ching*) A bow that is stretched to its fullest capacity may certainly snap. A sword that is tempered to its very sharpest may easily be broken.

KNEEPAD

"Active" R & R Warning Signs

SYSTEMIC

Irritability, depression

Loss of drive

Loss of appetite

Elevated morning resting heart (pulse) rate

Sleep disturbance

LOCAL

Persistent muscle soreness

Overuse injury (tennis elbow, rotator cuff injury, jumper's knee, stress fractures)

Drop in performance

Unexplained fatigue

occasional bout with sleep disturbance (including snoring, a sign of low-quality sleep), light exercise an hour before bedtime is a natural soporific (aka sleep remedy).

The lowdown on your knee fitness program is the same as that for any other exercise program: Gains in strength, flexibility, durability, and balance happen in your "down" time. So take a day, or even two, off, but stay active in other ways and make proper nutrition and sleep a priority.

ACTIVE EATING

For every pound you carry, your hip and knee think it's 5 (or more, depending on your type of activity) because of load stresses, so if you're 10 pounds overweight, it feels like 50 to your frame! Small amounts of extra weight are amplified across your knees, hips, and ankles. Excess pounds in your frame cause and accelerate damage, and hamper recovery from injury; they strain connective tissue, grind joints, and play a role in arthritis and other inflammation throughout your body.

The good news about poundage is that it works both ways—if you lose 5 pounds, your frame thinks you lost 25. That's a pretty good deal when you think about it, and it is why even small amounts of weight loss have been shown to lessen the progression of knee arthritis. But losing weight is one thing; keeping it off is quite another, and that's the primary drawback of otherwise excellent diet programs. They simply do not emphasize enough the critical ingredient in any diet: exercise.We're all too busy in our daily lives and sedentary as a rule in our leisure time (albeit with the best intentions to work out regularly "someday"), and wrestling with a diet is often enough on our "plates."

KNEEPAD

Sweet Dreams

No caffeine after lunch, and no major meal within 2 hours of bedtime.

Leave your work at work!

Invest in a good, comfortable mattress.

Read just before bedtime—no TV.

Meditate, don't medicate.

Whether or not you're overweight, I'm here to tell you that "someday" must be today because of the way your metabolism works. It was programmed way back in our evolution as a survival mechanism: If you diet and significantly cut back on calories consumed, the body senses starvation and plays a nasty trick on you: It starts to cannibalize muscle first, not fat. Muscles use a lot of calories, so loss of muscle mass lowers your metabolic rate. Thus, you're more vulnerable to gaining weight because of the lower metabolic rate (your internal furnace thermostat set point) that occurs when you lose muscle. You can short-circuit this vicious cycle with muscle building and toning, something I rarely, if ever, see addressed in weight-loss discussions and programs.

Complicating matters is the fact that you will gradually lose muscle and weaken your frame as you age. That's why we're prone to weight gain as we get older. So, everyone, no matter how heavy or how old, has to exercise, and their programs must include some sort of resistance training to build and/or maintain total body musculature. It maintains and builds bones and tendons in addition to muscle, and that's what helps keep any excess weight off the frame. With every bit of muscle you add, you raise your metabolic rate and burn more calories, even if you're just sitting around doing nothing.

As for a weight-loss diet, the primary factor is calorie control. Science tells us that a pound is equivalent to 3,500 calories, so if your goal is to lose a pound a week, calorie intake must be reduced by 500 calories each day. Most rapid weight-loss programs deprive the body of important nutrients, and the "rapid" weight that is lost is usually water and muscle. Not good! The goal is to lose fat and get leaner. Don't look at the scale—look at yourself in the mirror. As a famous bodybuilder once told me, "If you can't flex it, lose it." I don't think you have to go that far, but you get the message.

Now that you know that 3,500 calories equals 1 pound, it's a matter of calculating the number of calories you consume over a week, and that's not all that tough to do when we consider the almost-universal labeling nowadays. So keep a running tab of *every* calorie you put into your mouth over 7 days, without changing your usual eating routine. Whatever that number turns out to be, divide it by seven, subtract 500, and that's your daily calorie allotment that guarantees you'll lose weight. (I'll let you in on a little secret: Your 500-calorie reduction doesn't have to come solely from giving up some food. That's a good thing because if you're like me, you cherish every bite you take and might have a real tough time doing without some favorites. Watch your choice of beverages. Stick with water most of the time and cut out any sweet drinks, which are loaded with "naked" calories. Also, exercise of any kind burns calories in varying degree; 20 minutes of walking makes about 50 calories disappear, 20 minutes of vigorous gardening lops off 75, and the same time spent doing strenuous aerobics burns 150 or more.)

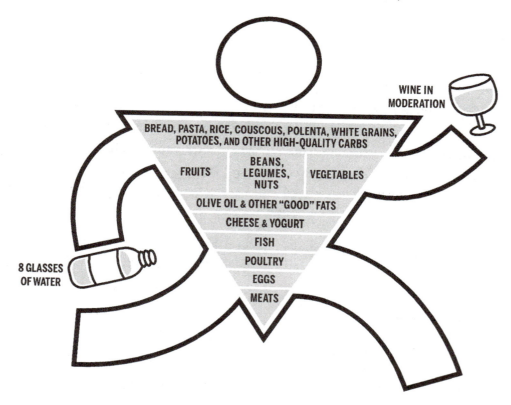

WINE IN MODERATION

BREAD, PASTA, RICE, COUSCOUS, POLENTA, WHITE GRAINS, POTATOES, AND OTHER HIGH-QUALITY CARBS

FRUITS

BEANS, LEGUMES, NUTS

VEGETABLES

OLIVE OIL & OTHER "GOOD" FATS

CHEESE & YOGURT

FISH

POULTRY

8 GLASSES OF WATER

EGGS

MEATS

JOINT DISCUSSION

Let's "chew" on food labels for a moment because they provide a wealth of vital information in addition to telling us the number of calories per serving of a food. Pay careful attention to the facts that calories are *per serving* and that there is a specific quantity of servings in the package that is listed right at the top of the label. So if you eat a bag of peanuts that contains three servings, and there are 100 calories per serving, you just consumed 300 calories, not 100.

Next, the total fat category is subdivided into saturated fat and trans fats (what's left after you subtract those two from total fat is usually the fat that is good for you). Stay completely away from trans fats and save saturated fat for a rare, special treat.

Most people should stay under 300 milligrams of cholesterol per day, the next label category; if you have heart issues or you were told your cholesterol is high, keep it below 200 milligrams. Moving down the label, the U.S. Recommended Dietary Allowance (RDA) for sodium is 2,400 milligrams, but research is pushing that number lower, toward the 1,600 milligram RDA in the United Kingdom. The RDA for potassium is 3,500 milligrams (a banana has about 400 milligrams; a cup of lima beans is close to 1,000 milligrams).

The all-important total carbohydrates category, subdivided into dietary fiber and sugars, is next. Very few among us get the 25 grams of fiber per day that is optimum for weight and blood glucose control, so hone in on that number when you weigh options on the shelf. Official U.S. guidelines advise a maximum of 40 grams of refined sugar per 2,000 calories, but try to cut that in half. (And note that "refined sugar" isn't just table sugar; it is also the kind that is in a wide range of processed foods such as breakfast cereal, so be "sweet" on this label tidbit.)

Last but not least are the protein and vitamin categories. The RDA for protein is 0.8 gram per kilogram (2.2 pounds) of body weight, and that is between 40 grams and 70 grams per day for most people. If you're pregnant or in the older crowd, you'll need a little more (consult your physician), and a 50 percent increase in your daily protein intake is recommended if you train hard. Most of us don't get enough protein in our daily diets. Look for high-quality protein sources and even supplement with a shake if needed. As for vitamins? Get as many and as much of them in your food as you can, and supplement when needed.

The labels for any food items that contain peanuts, lactose, and other ingredients that can cause severe allergic reactions will include that information as well. (My daughter Emily is allergic to peanuts, so she learned as a youngster to scan the labels of any foods she wasn't familiar with, and this has helped her become a nutrition guru at a very young age. She often has me put back certain things as she reminds me of what's on the label. Thank you, Emily!)

Proper nutrition is not so much about any one thing you eat as it is about getting used to what labels tell you and thinking about what you are putting into your body each day. If labels are a case of TMI for you, some nutritionists will gladly go on a field trip to the local supermarket with you to give you a "healthy" course on how to use them. That's what sports nutritionist Jeanie Subach does routinely for some players on the Philadelphia Eagles, Philadelphia Flyers, and Philadelphia 76ers. If they can do it, so can you.

There really isn't any magic involved with slimming down. It has nothing to do with a narrow focus on low carbs, all protein, good fats, or the new fad that either starves you or bores you to tears. It's about watching what you eat and taking advantage of the excellent nutrition in all food groups. I recommend the Mediterranean diet because it has everything you need and never bores the taste buds or the stomach, and it's great for your frame with all of its natural antioxidant and anti-inflammatory ingredients. There are others that are balanced with good carbs, friendly fats, and anti-inflammatory foods, so eat whatever you like—up to your limit and in proportion with the FrameWork Pyramid that maximizes grains and minimizes meat and eggs.

YOUR FRAMEWORK TRAINING TABLE

If you are what you just ate, you will be what you eat from now on. Again, you can choose what you eat, but you must choose wisely; you must include in your diet every major food group and every color of the rainbow. I'll leave the specifics about a menu up to you, but I have some general guidelines that will help you to maximize nutritional value.

- A good rule of thumb is to allocate 20 percent of your diet to protein, 15 percent

KNEEPAD

CALORIE BURN per HOUR

Walking—150

Housework—160

Gardening—225

Doubles tennis—350

Aerobics—450

Hiking—500

Light jogging—500

Swimming—500

Singles tennis—550

Power walking—600

Squash—650

Running—700

Water polo—700

to polyunsaturated fats, 10 percent to monounsaturated fats, and 55 percent to good carbs. When you make your choices from these categories, give the nod every time to the ones highest in fiber content.

■ Muscles require amino acids, those protein building blocks, and protein needs increase with age because of its associated muscle loss. Protein is always necessary to replenish muscle fibers, and yet protein is not as well absorbed into your system as you get older. The fact is, young or old, most of us do not take in enough protein. Why? Because we've all been cutting way back on red meat and eggs to reduce the risk of cardiovascular disease, and we haven't substituted enough of the better protein choices to make up the difference. Look for lean protein: chicken and turkey without the skin and salt (and hold the mayo, too), wild salmon, trout, herring, anchovies, and sardines, or soy if you're a vegetarian. Mix in more brown rice, beans, and lentils to make up any protein shortfall.

■ We've all been warned about the dangers associated with butter, cheese, cream, and whole milk, but make sure some of your menu choices include good fats. The medical literature is peppered with studies that confirm the efficacy of the omega-3 fatty acids in olive oil, oily fish, nuts, and seeds—staples of the Mediterranean diet. They're a boon to cardiovascular health,

JOINT DISCUSSION

I once had the privilege of spending an afternoon with Martina Navratilova. It was a small group tennis clinic that also allowed plenty of informal discussion. Martina is a real inspiration, and was one of the very first athletes to really focus on exercise training and nutrition to improve her sports performance, and ultimately her health. When I asked her about her early focus on nutrition, she quipped, "What you put in is what you get out." That's not just true for elite athletes like Martina, but also for you and me.

but they come with an advisory: Fats are extremely high in calories—200 in only a ¼ cup of some nuts, for example—so measure quantities very carefully. The upside is that a small amount goes a long way toward curbing your appetite. (Try a couple of tablespoons of hummus with half of a whole wheat pita or a sliced banana with some flaxseed sprinkled on it as an appetizer or snack and see for yourself.)

■ Good diets eliminate the carbs that aren't good for us—fried potatoes, white bread, white rice, sugar—but the best diet is loaded with carbs that fuel your frame while they fill your stomach—whole grains, leafy vegetables, fruit, and seeds. You don't have to totally give up bread and pasta; just make them a special treat or make sure they have the right (whole grain) ingredients, and, yes, you can indulge in the nutrition-rich potato—preferably boiled, steamed, or baked. Remember: The main fuel of choice for Olympic athletes is carbs. It really makes no sense to me when individuals who want to get fit and look better cut out carbs completely. For them I have two words: Michael Phelps. When training, this young super-athlete consumes more than 12,000 carb-loaded calories a day!

KNEEPAD

Good Carbs

Whole grain bread, cereal, pasta

Brown rice, couscous, chickpeas, lentils

Oat bran

Leafy vegetables

Seeds (pumpkin, sesame, sunflower, flax)
Fruit (especially pineapple, grapefruit, cherries, unsweetened strawberries, peaches, and cantaloupe)

KNEEPAD

Friendly Fats

Polyunsaturated

Safflower, sunflower, corn, soybean oils

Walnuts

Oily fish

Monounsaturated

Extra-virgin olive oil and canola oil

Avocados

Peanuts, hazelnuts, almonds, cashews

■ Next on the FrameWork menu are foods that minimize inflammation and oxidation. It's no coincidence that the protein, good carbs, and friendly fats discussed above not only provide the right, balanced nutrition, they also decrease inflammatory and cell-destructive reactions in your body. You might have noticed that junk food, fried food, saturated and partially hydrogenated fats, bakery goods, and sweets were nowhere to be found in the diet recommendations here. These food selections should be avoided like the plague because of the systemic havoc they wreak in your body. They promote the enemy, inflammation, which can be destructive to both your heart and your frame. It is no wonder that the Mediterranean diet is recommended for individuals with arthritis because it is packed with anti-inflammatory nutrients.

■ Accent your menu with a wide variety of spices that don't add calories to your plate and make your food tastier as they deliver antioxidation and anti-inflammation support.

KNEEPAD

The Rainbow of Nutrition

Red: Tomatoes, red peppers, pink grapefruit, watermelon, cherries

Purple: Blueberries, plums, beets, eggplant, red cabbage

Reddish orange: Carrots, mangoes, cantaloupe, winter squash, sweet potatoes

Yellow/orange: Peaches, papayas, nectarines, pineapples

Yellow/green: Spinach, corn, green peas, avocados, honeydew melon

Green: Broccoli, Brussels sprouts, cabbage, kale, bok choy

White/green: Garlic, onions, leeks, celery, asparagus, pears, green grapes

Last, but not least, is a word about hydration. Water makes digestion possible; it is a solvent for nutrients and transports them everywhere. It assists muscle contraction and serves as a shock absorber all over your body. Water regulates your body temperature and eliminates waste products. And, for all you weight battlers out there, it fills you up and neutralizes food cravings.

Your blood is 90 percent water, your brain is 85 percent water, your muscles are 72 percent water, and your skin is 71 percent water. A water deficiency shows up as reduced mental acuity, fatigue, wrinkled skin, or the muscle cramps that both professional athletes and regular folks get sometimes when engaging in sports. If you feel plum tuckered out, have a headache or eye strain, or sore muscles in your neck and back, it might have nothing at all to do with overwork and stress—it just might be a serious lack of aqua.

Bottom line? You need to drink 2 quarts of water every day. As it is with fiber, however, few among us consume that much. So be like one of those people we see all around who have a water bottle in their hand, cup holder, or carryall, or on their desk. (Drinks that contain caffeine don't count—caffeine is a diuretic that drains body fluid. If you've had your "fill" of water, try grape, cherry, acai, goji, or pomegranate juice; teas that don't contain caffeine; or smoothies made in a blender using fruit, ice, and low-fat yogurt.)

SUPPLEMENTAL NUTRITIONAL ADVICE

Even if you eat all the best things all the time, your gastrointestinal system is inefficient—it can't extract all of the good nutrients from the food you ingest. That, coupled with taste preferences that may inadvertently be causing you to miss out on something your frame needs, is why every diet must include some basic over-the-counter (OTC) supplements. (Beware, you bargain shoppers out there: Unlike with. pharmaceutical-grade drugs, there is currently no government regulation to ensure that supplements meet label claims. Many companies use foreign suppliers whose ingredients have less-than-advertised potency, and some use additional substances not on the label that could be quite harmful to you, especially if you are taking any prescription medication. Even if a supplement company meets label claims in terms of amount or dosage of ingredients, that is only one side of the coin. Bioavailability—or how readily the substance can get into your system—can vary dramatically depending on the quality of the ingredient and the supply source. So it is not only quantity, but also quality where many supplements fall short. This is especially true in the world of joint supplements, where studies using independent testing have shown that even among the top 10 selling brands, quality and quantity of ingredients can vary drastically. Some brands are very inconsistent in terms of what's actually inside, and some have little or no active ingredient—that is, they are selling blanks! This is why I can't say enough that brand really matters—do your research and buy only from reputable manufacturers that conform to strict codes regarding product quality and labeling. The best companies earn the United States Pharmacopeia [USP] seal of approval.) Interestingly, in Europe the joint supplements glucosamine, chondroitin sulfate, and ASU are all available by prescription only and are thus under greater scrutiny and quality control.

In addition to a broad-spectrum multivitamin, a program that buttresses your diet and bolsters your frame covers three vital

KNEEPAD

Use Salutary Spices Liberally

Top 10 Antioxidant Condiments

Turmeric

Cinnamon

Oregano

Cloves

Parsley

Basil

Cumin

Sage

Mustard seed

Marjoram

Top 10 Anti-Inflammation Condiments

Hot chile peppers

Ginger

Curry powder

Black pepper

Rosemary

Basil

Cloves

Garlic

Parsley

Onion

areas: bone/connective tissue support (see "Over-the-Counter Supplement Remedies for Arthritis" in Step 2 on page 48), antioxidant protection, and inflammation control. (Check "Supplement Your Frame" on the opposite page for a detailed list.)

Digestive inefficiencies also explain in part those hunger pangs we get now and then. One trick of a diet you can stick to is to split your daily protein allowance over two or three meals; protein takes longer to break down, so you feel full longer. Another trick is to allocate 20 to 40 percent of your daily calorie allowance to healthy snacks. Many people find having multiple, smaller "meals" spread throughout the day keeps them satisfied and lessens the urge to binge at regular mealtimes. This approach also tends to keep blood sugar and insulin levels more stable throughout the day. Get in the habit of having a resealable plastic bag with some goodies (seeds, raisins, celery, carrots, broccoli, grapes) handy so you don't end up with a soda or candy bar to satisfy a craving with 300 or more empty calories.

Yes, weight management and healthy nutrition come down to the choices you make every day about what you will put into your mouth—both quantity and quality. You'll either increase your fat, your blood sugar, your weight, and

inflammatory reactions in your muscles and joints, or reduce them with the help of Mother Nature. Acquire better food habits and make better choices: extra-virgin olive oil and vinegar instead of Caesar salad dressing; teas and unsweetened juices instead of soda that blocks calcium absorption because of its phosphorus content; dark honey or stevia instead of sugar; mustard instead of mayo; spices instead of salt; fresh food prepared fast instead of fast food. (And don't forget to grab a cup of water every chance you get.)

Eat well and have fun doing it. It's a great way to extend your frame's warranty.

MIND MATTERS

Sports medicine doctors know that taking psychological issues into consideration is important when dealing with orthopedic problems and injuries. And yet history has shown that many, if not most, of us aren't very good at doing anything about them. There are times when I walk into an examination room and before I even know what the patient's issue is, I have a feeling, a sixth sense, that I won't be able to help that person. I know that the right diagnosis and treatment won't be enough to get that person better because there are emotional or other

KNEEPAD

Supplement Your Frame

Bone/Connective Tissue Support

Glucosamine/chondroitin sulfate (1,500 milligrams/1,200 milligrams)*

Calcium (1,200 milligrams)

Vitamin D3 (1,000 IU)

L-arginine (1,600 milligrams)

L-glutamine (1,000 milligrams)

Avocado-soybean unsaponifiables (300 milligrams)*

Methylsulfonylmethane, or MSM (3,000 milligrams)

Antioxidant Protection

Pycnogenol, a pine bark extract (100 milligrams)

Coenzyme Q10, or CoQ10 (50 milligrams)

Grapeseed extract (100 milligrams) with resveratrol (20 milligrams)

L-glutathione, reduced form (100 milligrams)

Green tea extract (epigallocatechin-3 gallate or EGCG)

Tart cherry juice

Resveratrol** (red grapes and red wine)

Omega-3s

Inflammation Control

Glucosamine/chondroitin sulfate (1,500 milligrams/1,200 milligrams)*

Avocado-soybean unsaponifiables (300 milligrams)*

Green tea extract (epigallocatechin-3 gallate or EGCG)

Curcumin (400 milligrams)

Quercetin (500 milligrams)

S-adenosylmethionine, or SAM-e (800 milligrams)

Willow bark (1,600 milligrams)

Gamma linolenic acid, or GLA (250 milligrams)

Flaxseed (2,000 milligrams)

Tart cherry juice

Bromelain (pineapple)

Omega-3s

*I recommend the Cosamin DS and Cosamin ASU formulations from Nutramax Labs (nutramaxlabs.com).

**I recommend Bioforte from Biotivia (biotivia.com).

psychosocial issues involved. That "baggage" hasn't been checked.

Orthopedic specialists are aware of the importance of a patient's mind "frame." We've seen the same studies every other doctor has that unequivocally connect stress with immune dysfunction and disease, but we haven't connected all the dots on how to help patients who are stressed out. Mind and body tend to be seen as two completely different and completely separate realms. We, as surgeons, all too often just deal with the physical; we don't get patients to the right person, or incorporate a team approach, or, perhaps most important of all, call on them to help themselves emotionally. The result is suboptimal healing and/or recovery, and recurrent frame-related (or other) ailments.

That's beginning to change in a big way. Psychoneuroimmunology (PNI) is a medical discipline, still in its formative stages, that was established to clarify the complex hormonal and biochemical triggers that alter the immune response and other physiological systems. These triggers either allow your mind and central nervous system to give you a boost, or they set off a downward spiral. It's been documented beyond question that stress plays a major role in both acute and chronic pain.

Helen Flanders Dunbar, MD, said, "It's not a question of whether an illness is physical or emotional, but h ow much of each." Simply stated, if we ignore the emotional side, we're not going to be as successful as we could be in getting people better. In my experience, a significant number of doctors fail to appreciate this. So we see more tests, more surgeries, more utilization of our already strained health-care system—not always to the advantage of the patient.

Stress, anxiety, depression, and other emotional issues are often the elephant in the corner of the room that all are ignoring. Your doctor might see it, but he or she might not be comfortable dealing with it. You need to be honest with yourself and bring it up, even if it is only a potential factor. It may be one of the keys to getting you better and/or avoiding unnecessary treatment.

When it comes to psychological distress, clearly there is a wide range of severity. Anyone who is affected daily (causing a slip in work life or relationships) by any mind issue must seek professional help. If there are psychosocial issues in play in your case, talk with your doctor about possible interventions. I've heard, and I believe, that broken bodies are easier to heal than broken minds. Addressing the mind is an important step toward optimal healing and recovery, and it's a big part of the FrameWork program.

STARVE WHATEVER IT IS THAT'S EATING YOU

Doctors aren't the only ones not doing enough when it comes to mind frame—everyone bears some responsibility for how he or she feels and how that affects overall health. You may not be able to do much about the circumstances that weigh upon you, but you sure can acknowledge they exist (don't bury your head in the sand about them), and you sure can do a lot to combat them.

■ RELAXATION BREATHING

Unconsciously, most of us take shallow breaths all day long, and that is the rule when we are in pain or in an excited or agitated state, which actually produces or exacerbates stress.

The following routine to calm you down is so simple that you can do it anywhere, anytime, and it's something you should do a few times every day and whenever you are experiencing discomfort or pain.

1. Find a quiet place and get comfortable. Try to relax and let go of tension in your body.

2. Notice your regular breathing—feel your breath expanding your lungs, then emptying from your lungs.

3. Take deeper breaths and notice how the infusion of additional oxygen clears your head. Focus exclusively on this, driving everything else from your mind.

4. Take even deeper breaths slowly through your nose. Hold for 1 to 2 seconds. Release the air through your mouth while relaxing your entire body. Repeat three times.

5. Breathe normally through your nose three times, focusing on the oxygen coming into your body and thinking

KNEEPAD

De-Stress

Relaxation Breathing and Meditation

ID Your Stress Buttons

Open Your Relief Valve

Talk It Out

Soothe Yourself

Think Positive

Eat Right and Stay Hydrated

Exercise

Sleep Tight

about it expanding your chest, entering your bloodstream, and circulating from your forehead to your toes.

6. Continue taking slow, deep breaths through your nose, but now let your belly expand so that you're breathing with your diaphragm. When your lungs are full, hold the breath for 2 seconds. (Until you get this deeper breathing down, place your palms on your abdominal area and actually feel your abdomen expand.)

7. Release the breath slowly through your mouth and exhale until your lungs feel completely empty—contract your belly to force out every last air molecule. (If your palms are still on your abdomen, you will feel it deflate and slightly tighten at the end when all of your air is exhaled.) Wait 2 seconds.

8. Repeat the cycle three times starting with step 4.

▨ ID YOUR STRESS BUTTONS

There are certain things—at home, at work, at school, even at play—that set your mind and body racing. You usually know what they are (if not, you need to start figuring it out), and you know when they kick in. What you might not know is that you can train yourself to switch off your brain. As soon as one of

these things occurs, you can make the conscious decision to distract your mind with a more pleasant or innocuous thought. Practice this—it works.

▨ OPEN YOUR RELIEF VALVE

You also know what calms you down, what distracts you from whatever worries you have and gets you into the psychological state called flow. Exercise, tennis, and juggling work for me; whatever works for you—a leisurely stroll, model building, poker playing, listening to your playlist, frolicking with the kids—should be brought to the fore whenever you need to let off steam. And, although you can't find it in any anatomy book, your "tickle bone" is an essential part of your frame—find it, and laugh your cares away every now and then.

▨ TALK IT OUT

Keeping things bottled up can and will backfire with physical and emotional consequences. Talk to a friend, a significant other, or your doctor. Let things out; it helps. In *FrameWork for the Lower Back* I cited a recent study published in the *Archives of Internal Medicine* that showed participation in an e-mail discussion group was enough to help reduce pain and disability in individuals with chronic lower back pain. There's no reason to think it wouldn't work for knee (or mind) pain as well. So please talk or chat or text your way to better health.

SOOTHE YOURSELF

There is a host of things that pacify just like Mom used to do (or still does, if you're fortunate to still have her with you). Listening to waves at the seashore or staring into a fire (and other repetitive nature sounds and images); taking a long, hot bath; massage; yoga; meditation; tai chi; progressive muscle relaxation, or PMR (see page 106, and combine it with Relaxation Breathing on page 103); and drinking hot tea or water with lemon all have remarkable salutary effects. Take every opportunity you can to nurture your mind frame.

THINK POSITIVE

It might not be in your nature to be optimistic, but its proven benefits are so huge that it pays to learn to suspend your disbelief or cynicism. Pick up one or a couple of the bestsellers on this

JOINT DISCUSSION

Right before every intense surgical session, I set aside a few moments to be alone with my breathing. It's something I learned with exposure over the years to martial arts, yoga, and meditation that helps me "cool" my systems. A little time—less than 2 minutes, actually—focusing solely on the air entering and leaving my body, and I'm ready for anything that lies ahead. I'm relaxed, and my concentration is heightened.

topic and adopt the approaches and techniques that are comfortable for you.

Guided imagery (used for centuries by yogis to control heart rate and body temperature) is a form of positive thinking. Studies have shown that an aquarium in a room can lower blood pressure and that conjuring a tranquil place or activity in your mind can have the same effect. Stay with the image, make it real, and don't be surprised if your tension eases.

Along with the above approaches, here are a few others to keep stress in check.

Eat right. (Food affects mood, as anyone who has witnessed a child after a sugar binge could tell you.)

- Hydrate, hydrate, hydrate. (We've discussed how a lack of water can strain your eyes, neck, and back—is it a surprise that these add to overall tension?)

- Stick to an exercise program and get proper sleep.

There are a lot of proven stress reducers to choose from here, but don't let that increase your anxiety. The only "must learn" strategy is Relaxation Breathing because its calming effect not only cuts tension but also prepares your frame for exercise. As for the rest, again, choose wisely and incorporate everything that's appropriate to your circumstance and preference.

KNEEPAD

Progressive Muscle Relaxation (PMR)

In succession:

- Clench and unclench your jaw.

- Shrug your shoulders.

- Make a tight fist and release it.

- Tense and untense your arms, torso, pelvic area, and legs.

- Feel the tension leave your muscles and body.

ACTIVE KNEES, STEP-BY-STEP

If you are to extend the warranty on your hinges to the fullest, you have to have a healthy lifestyle, balanced fitness, and a mind that's in good shape. In other words: overall health. Paying attention to these approaches will get you there. If you want to delve into these topics in greater detail, I refer you to my original FrameWork book, *FrameWork: Your 7-Step Program for Healthy Muscles, Bones, and Joints.*

When you've got overall health, you minimize the chances for knee problems and maximize the benefits of taking the next step, which strengthens your hinges with targeted exercise. As a knee specialist, I have seen far too many weak, damaged, or injured knees exert a domino effect, negatively impacting individuals' entire lives. And this doesn't have to be the case.

If your knees are creaky now, they'll quiet down; if you're a recreational sport enthusiast, you'll play better; if you just want to get out of your car and climb a flight of stairs without grabbing a knee or a handrail for assistance, it can be so. Just turn the page and start a whole new chapter in an active life.

SHAPELY KNEES

Most of the patients I see are committed to regular exercise, but approximately 80 percent of adults need a modification to their program because it overworks or underworks one or more vulnerable or potentially vulnerable frame part. From the most tentative participant to the most seasoned workout fanatic, something just isn't right. If they stick to the "generic" program, not the one customized for *their* frame, they will certainly get into trouble, if they haven't already. The satisfaction I get from their efforts is tempered by the worry that they'll injure themselves and discontinue one of the very best things they can do for their health—being active for life.

A major scientific study has shown that one-third of exercisers had to drop out of a very conservative, medically supervised fitness program because a musculoskeletal ailment—a frame injury—cropped up. The researchers were surprised, but I wasn't. So if problems can result under tight supervision, imagine what could happen if you don't go about things in the right way. Your regimen might be great on the merits, but it might not be great for *your* frame.

Does it make much sense to sign up for a marathon if you can't walk to the corner store without difficulty? Of course not. Likewise, it isn't prudent to vigorously train your knees if your body and mind aren't in tune for that exercise, if you aren't fit in general. If you have an issue specifically with your knees, it is especially important to have your program appropriately customized to keep you on the field or at the gym—and out of my office. And there is no getting around the previous step that must be a prelude to the programs designed for your hinges.

Before we get to those, a couple of reminders are critical.

■ Never embark upon a new exercise routine without a phone call to your primary physician and any other appropriate health-care provider, especially someone who is involved in the care of the body part that the routine targets, to disclose your intent. Before you make the call, answer the questions in the Physical Activity Readiness Questionnaire (see opposite page), which was developed in Canada to help individuals determine if they need to see a doctor before starting an exercise program. If you answer yes to any of the questions, be sure to mention this to your doctor, who will almost always then schedule an appointment for a thorough examination. If you honestly answered no to all of the PARQ questions, you can be reasonably sure that you can start becoming much more physically active. (The American College of Sports Medicine, ACSM, offers a more comprehensive pre-exercise screening based on your age, health status, current or past symptoms, and medical risk factors. If you have a sedentary lifestyle and/or are older than 50, I strongly recommend an ACSM-type assessment.)

■ Slow, controlled movement, not bouncing to and fro, is the cornerstone of safe and effective exercise routines. And keep in mind there is significant benefit from both concentric (up) and eccentric (down) motion. Optimal balanced muscle growth and development require attention to both phases of the lift, up and down. Also, the exercises to come will be more effective if you use a mindfulness technique whereby you stay focused and concentrate on the muscles being called upon during the movements.

IN THE STARTING BLOCKS

Have you ever noticed how competitive runners do some last-minute stretches and take a few deep breaths right before they get into position for a race? I have, and as a physician for professional athletes for many years, I have had the opportunity to arrive at the stadium hours before a sporting match begins, and I can tell you that athletes devote an extensive amount of time to preparing their bodies for what's to come, executing all of the movements required for their sport at reduced speed.

Regardless of the sport or recreational exercise, your frame has to be properly prepared if you want to perform better—and avoid injury. Before you dash out the door in

KNEEPAD

Physical Activity Readiness Questionnaire (PARQ)

1. Has your doctor ever said that you have a heart condition and that you should only do physical activity recommended by a doctor?
2. Do you feel pain in your chest when you do physical activity?
3. In the past month, have you had chest pain when you were not doing physical activity?
4. Do you lose your balance because of dizziness, or do you ever lose consciousness?
5. Do you have a bone or joint problem (for example, back, hip, or knee) that could be made worse by a change in your physical activity?
6. Is your doctor currently prescribing drugs (for example, water pills) for your blood pressure or heart condition?
7. Do you know of any other reason why you should not do physical activity?

KNEEPAD

Proper Warmup

- Relaxation breathing
- Light cardio
- S-t-r-e-t-c-h

running attire, pick up a racquet or golf club, hit the gym, or engage in the targeted exercise that follows, devote a couple of minutes to the relaxation breathing routine outlined in the previous step and to the other two activities—a light cardio warmup and stretching—that ensure a healthy workout.

Cardio Warmup

You've got to get your blood moving before you exercise. And the more in shape you get, the more important warming up is because your body is capable of doing more and will tax its frame members more. (Remember, warming up is different than stretching. Warming up brings blood to your muscles, lubricates your joints, and allows your musculoskeletal tissues to behave more elastically and thus be less vulnerable to injury.)

Two to three minutes of jumping jacks,

cycling, power walking, jogging, or marching in place is all it takes. The key is to break a light sweat; do it every time to avoid injury and get the most out of your knee exercises.

S-T-R-E-T-C-H

This is a great idea anytime; it's indispensable prior to a workout. For those of you who are strung particularly tight, try to stretch every day and follow the 3 x 30 stretching routine whereby you hold each stretch for 30 seconds and do it 3 times. For athletes or those involved in sports, additional dynamic stretches (such as arm swings and other joint rotations) can also be helpful and should be incorporated. Also, consider taking up yoga

JOINT DISCUSSION

Tennis is my passion, and if I didn't do the following routine religiously, I'd be on the sidelines a lot more.

- 30 jumping jacks
- Jogging in place
- Rotational twists
- Side bends
- Toe-touching
- Deep knee bends (I have to hold on to something because of a cranky knee, and I can't get all the way down.)
- Forearm and calf stretching
- To awaken muscle memory, tennis-specific movement patterns done while holding my racquet: windmills, low-intensity service motion, and practice swings (starting in slow motion and gradually increasing the pace, all while using the visualization technique to hone my shots)
- Gentle volleying from midcourt for a couple of minutes

I spend a scant 5 minutes off the court and about the same on it. In less than 10 minutes, I'm good to go.

KNEEPAD

Knee health starts on the floor and ends in the core.

and get a copy of *Stretching* by Bob Anderson (Shelter Publications), or my original *Frame-Work* book.

Remember: Your knees are connected to the rest of your frame, and every part must work in concert. You'll reap maximum reward with the following flexibility routines that should precede any frame workout (after you've broken a sweat with a cardio warmup, of course).

PROGRAM YOUR KNEES

If you've had knee surgery recently or you've got a balky knee, the Recovery and Injury-Specific Rehab and Exercise Programs on page 152 are where you should begin getting your hinges back in shape. But don't skip the Standard Knee Program that follows because that's what you'll be doing soon enough, when your knees are healthy or asymptomatic and you want to keep them that way.

The standard program works all of the primary knee muscles—quadriceps, hamstring, and calf—and the hip, pelvic, and core muscles that work in conjunction with them. It also gives the feet and ankles a biomechanical workout because their proprioception is a critical part of fine-tuned knee movement. This comprehensive exercise routine is divided into four categories:

- Flexibility
- Strength
- Core and More
- Neuromuscular Training

Start with the first exercise in each area and add the next one when you are comfortable enough to do so. For many of the specific body parts, I offer a variety of exercise options, including ones that can be done at home (with minimal, if any, equipment) or at the gym. Pick one or two that target each muscle group—no need to do them all. Don't worry if you can do only certain ones at the start, or if one area is problematical for you. Each person has a unique set of circumstances related to body weight, overall fitness, and health issues, and your frame will be introduced to exercises it hasn't experienced yet. There is no timetable for getting to all of them; just work steadily at your own pace while keeping the goal of being able to do all of them (hopefully someday) in mind.

STANDARD KNEE PROGRAM

The comprehensive routine that follows contains quite a number of individual exercises, but if you're a FrameWork veteran, you are already doing many of them. If you aren't, you'll find that once you get into the hang of a knee workout, it will be easy to incorporate into your regular non-aerobic workouts.

Don't fret if a piece of equipment isn't available or if you can't do every exercise at the start. If you go to a gym, you can find machines that will accomplish much of what we are recommending. If you work out at home, and want to use strength equipment, a single "multi" trainer like the Nautilus Freedom Trainer is perfect and takes up little room. All of the strength exercises can also be done with some simple, inexpensive portable items like elastic bands or tubing, and exercise balls that you can get from www.SPRI.com (see Additional Resources on page 194). Just keep in mind that if you don't work your hinges on a regular basis, you won't be getting the most out of your frame—and you'll be setting yourself up for problems down the road.

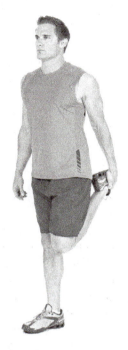

Standing Quadriceps Stretch

Keep your knees together at all times, resisting the temptation to allow your thigh to move outward. The body cheats two ways to allow you to get your foot to your buttock, and you should avoid these cheats. In the first cheat, to get your foot to your buttock, you spread your knees, abducting your hip; in the second cheat, you look downward and lean slightly forward, relaxing the front of your hip and upper quad. Both take away the effectiveness of the stretch.

Stand upright but use your right hand to support you (until you get really good at this and can balance without difficulty). Grab your left foot with your left hand and bring your heel up to your buttock, keeping your knees together at all times. Stand tall and don't lean forward at the waist or upper body. Hold for 10 seconds and repeat with your right hand and foot.

Advanced Version: If you can easily get your heel to your buttock, then increase the stretch by standing very tall, keeping your knees inward and touching. Next, pull back on your foot, extending your hip backward while staying tall and not leaning forward. Your knees should be pointing backward slightly.

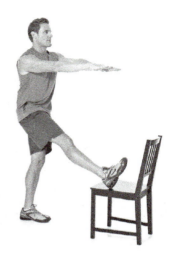

Figure 4 Hamstring Stretch

Sit on the floor in the figure 4 position with your left leg straight out, your foot pointing upward, and your ankle at a 90-degree angle. Sit tall (as if a string were pulling the top of your head toward the ceiling) and reach forward (like a walking zombie), with your index fingers touching side by side. While staying tall and keeping your chest high, slowly lean forward, keeping your left knee straight, and try to touch the wall (at the level of your eyes—that is, don't reach down toward your toes, but stay tall with good sitting posture). Hold for 20 seconds and then switch sides.

Alternate version: Rest your right heel on a chair or low staircase step, keeping your leg perfectly straight. Standing tall with your arms out forward, lean into the chair or staircase as far as you can go and hold for 10 to 20 seconds. Do not lean down and try to touch your toes. Repeat with your left leg.

Hamstring PNF alternative: Many individuals have difficulty with tight hamstrings. Proprioceptive neuromuscular facilitation (PNF) techniques have been used by therapists for almost any muscle group but seem to work particularly well with hamstrings. One PNF technique involves first contracting the muscle and then going immediately into a stretch. This temporarily short-circuits and fools the muscle. For the hamstring, start with your straight right leg on a chair or firm bench with the heel resting on the surface. Isometrically tighten your hamstring muscle by pulling down on your heel as if you were trying to press the top of the chair downward, keeping the leg straight or only slightly flexed. Hold this tightly for 10 seconds and feel the back of your thigh/hamstring to ensure it is tightening. Next, relax the muscle and immediately go into a hamstring stretch, holding for 30 seconds. Repeat 3 times on each side. (To avoid raising your blood pressure, be sure to breathe comfortably throughout this exercise, especially with the isometric muscle hold.)

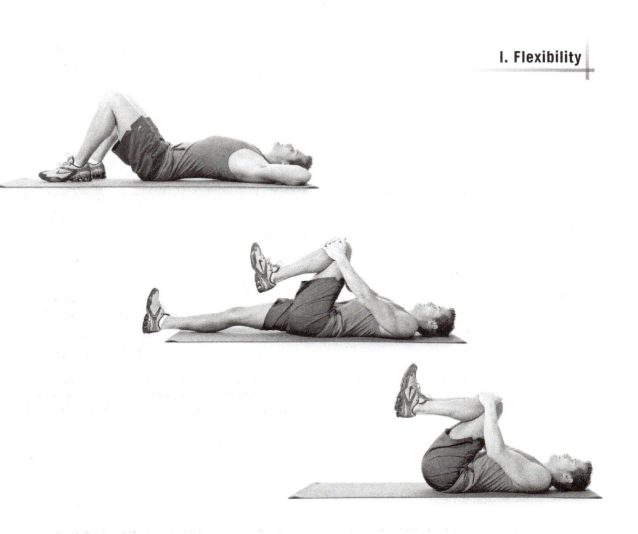

Knee-to-Chest

Lie on your back with your knees bent and feet flat on the floor. Pull your left leg/knee toward your chest with your hands behind the knee area (or in front if that is more comfortable); at the same time, straighten your right leg. Breathe gently and relax, keeping your head on the floor. Hold for 10 to 20 seconds. Repeat with the right leg. Next, pull both knees to your chest. Relax and hold for 10 to 20 seconds. (If you are comfortable with these static positions, you can add a slight rocking motion.) Repeat the sequence 3 or 4 times.

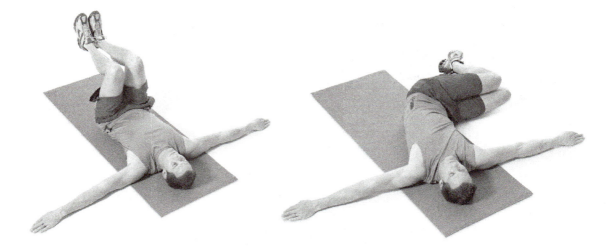

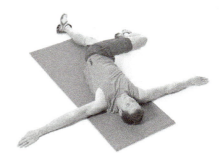

T-Roll

Lie on your back with your legs straight and your arms stretched out so that you form a T. Bring both knees up so that your hips and knees are flexed to 90 degrees. Keeping the palms of your hands, elbows, and shoulders on the floor (don't let them lift off), twist your torso and rotate your pelvis and knees so that your right knee is on the ground by your side, keeping your knees together. Hold for 5 to 7 seconds. Repeat on the opposite side. Repeat the sequence 2 times.

Alternate version: Keep your right leg straight while rotating your left leg over to the floor at your right. Repeat on the opposite side. Repeat the sequence twice.

Note: If your lower back and hips are tight, you may only be able to partially rotate and not have your knee reach the ground. Gradually try to improve how far you go.

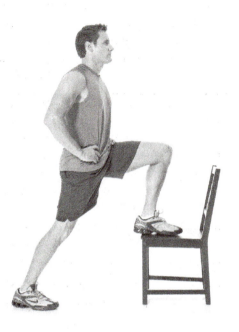

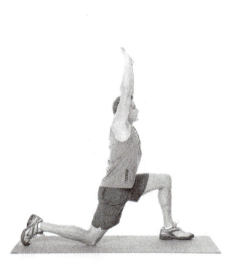

Psoas Stretch

Place your left foot flat on the top of a hard chair, stool, or step so that it's about 2 feet above the floor. Keep your right leg straight, with your foot pointing forward or slightly inward. Lean forward, keeping your back straight, until you feel a stretch in the front of your right hip. Hold for 20 seconds, and then alternate sides. Rest for a minute or two and repeat.

Alternate: Kneel on your right knee with your left leg out in front of your chest, and your left foot planted on the floor and pointing forward. Raise both arms over your head with your palms together. Lean your body forward until you feel a stretch in the front of your right hip and upper thigh. Hold for 20 seconds and then switch sides.

Note: This stretch can also be done with your arms relaxed at your sides, but the arms-up version gives a better stretch and improves posture. Keep your hands over your head, with your palms together. Reach as high as you can and stay tall with a straight spine.

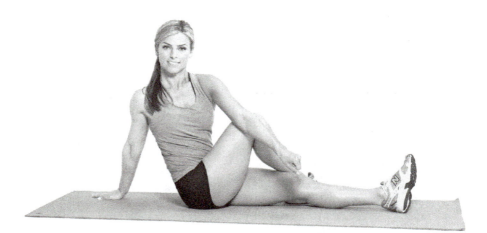

Pretzel ITB

Sit with your left leg straight out and your right foot crossed over and just to the outside of your left knee. Place the outer side of your left elbow on the outer side of your right knee and thigh. Use your left elbow to pull your right knee inward (to the left) and lock it there. You should feel a stretch in the right outer hip and thigh area.

Next, rotate your body so you are looking over your right shoulder as far as you can. (If you are in the center of the room, try to see the left corner behind you.)

Repeat on the opposite side.

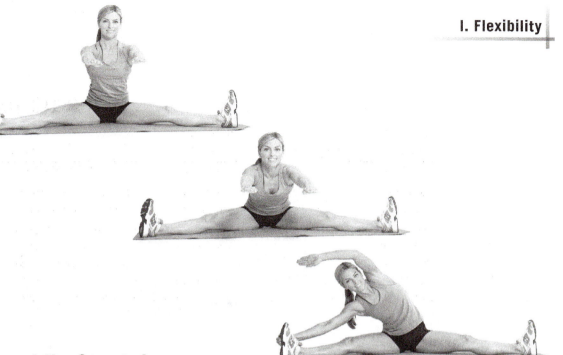

Straddle Stretch

Sit upright with your legs positioned out wide as far as comfortably possible. Keeping your back straight, slowly lean forward with your hands reaching straight out (not downward). You should feel the stretch in your inner thigh (adductor muscle) and hamstring area. Hold for 10 to 20 seconds and repeat 3 times.

Try to go a little wider with your legs as your flexibility improves. This is also a good stretch to do with a partner. Face each other and have your stretching partner (sitting in a similar position) place his or her feet on the inner side of your lower legs down near your ankle area. Your partner then holds your hands and gently assists pulling you forward for the stretch, while simultaneously keeping your legs abducted wide with his or her feet. (If you have hip arthritis, you will be limited in how wide your hips and legs will be able to go out, so don't force anything and stay within your comfort level.)

Advanced version: An alternate, more advanced version includes the straddle with a right and left bend.

Modification: A home or office alternative makes use of a staircase. Starting at the bottom of the steps, turn sideways so that your left leg is straight and the inner arch area of your left foot is resting on one of the lower steps. Pick a step that gives you a slight stretching sensation on the inner thigh. While holding this position, allow your right knee to drop down slightly, enhancing the stretch on the left inner thigh. Hold for 20 seconds. Repeat on the opposite side.

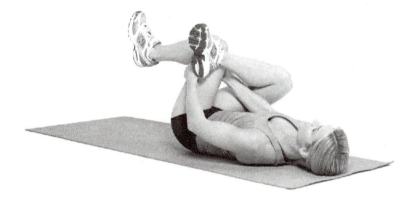

Piriformis Stretch

Lie on your back and flex both of your knees upward so your knees and hips are at 90-degree angles. Cross your right ankle over your left knee. Place your hands behind your left thigh and pull your right knee toward your chest. You should feel a stretch in the buttock and outer thigh area. Hold for 30 seconds and repeat on the opposite side.

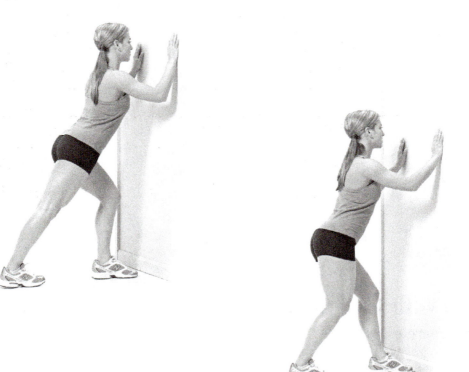

Calf Stretch

The calf muscle has two major components: the upper portion or gastrocnemius (which crosses the back of the knee) and the soleus or lower portion, which becomes your Achilles tendon behind your ankle. These components need to be stretched separately.

These stretches are good for the both the gastrocnemius and soleus muscles, the Achilles tendon, and the plantar fascia (arch) area. Doing it barefoot is best. Start with your knee straight, stretching the soleus (hold for 20 seconds), then bring your foot forward a little and do the flexed-knee version, which you will feel lower down. (An alternate stretch can be done off a step or machine by allowing your heel to drop.) Always keep your foot pointed straight ahead or preferably "pigeon-toed" inward a little. The cheat or mistake is to turn your foot outward a little, which allows your foot to roll into pronation, making this stretch easier, and thus less effective.

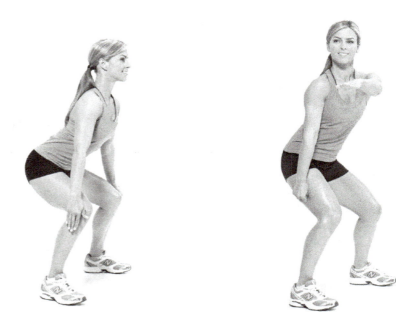

Horse with Ab Hollow

This is a great exercise that can be done several times per day. Done properly, it will build leg (quad) strength and endurance, and improve posture. Anyone with a background in the martial arts will attest to the importance of this one move, and it's a great idea to use the relaxation breathing technique (see page 103) while doing it. (If you have any knee restrictions or pain that prevents you from doing this exercise, try the Wall Seat on the opposite page instead.)

Start with your feet wider than shoulder-width apart and pointing forward. Stay tall, and keep your back and head straight and your abs tight as you begin to sink into a partial sitting position. Look straight ahead. Keep your knees outward, beyond your feet so that if you look down, your feet are pointing straight ahead on the inner side of your knees. Hold for 20 seconds, and try to build up to several minutes over time. Another alternative is to slowly move up and down from the Horse position to a full standing position while concentrating on keeping your abs straight and your pelvis stable.

Advanced modification: As you improve the length of time holding this position, you can add the side-reach modification, in which you twist your torso area and reach as far as possible to the left side with your right arm, then reach as far as possible to the right side with your left arm, and continue alternating sides.

Note: Ideally you should try to keep your back straight, with your shoulders more in line with your hips.

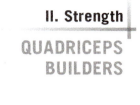

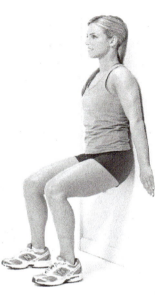

Wall Seat

Stand with your back to a wall about a foot or so away from it. Lean against the wall and do a modified Horse as your body allows, sliding down the wall one-quarter of the way at first. You should feel a burning sensation in the thigh muscle area (this is good) and not burning or pain in the kneecap area (not good). As you get stronger, you should gradually be able to go down farther. (If you feel pain under the kneecap, you are going too far. Sometimes there is a mid-range of discomfort, and you can actually go lower, beyond a comfortable position.)

If you have patellar pain syndrome with kneecap pain, then do a modified Horse or Wall Seat in the partial-sitting, partial-knee flexion position as your body allows. Also, do not step out as far and flex your knee only partially, that is, one-quarter of the way down. If you are unable to do this version, you will need to work on quad isometrics daily until you're able to do it. (For more information, see Patellar Pain Syndrome on page 159.)

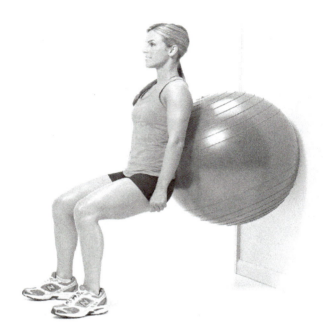

Horse on Ball against Wall

Get into position as for the Wall Seat but first put a stability ball between you and the wall. The ball should press against your middle or lower back when you're in the starting position, and rise to your mid to upper back as you flex downward. Hold this position for 60 seconds and increase the time as your legs get stronger.

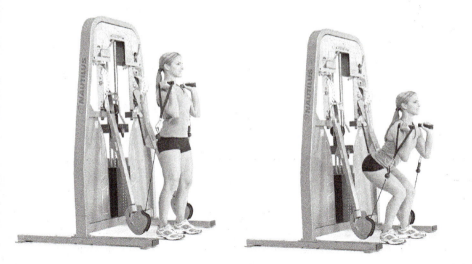

Squat/Leg Press
(3 variations with progressing challenge)

1. Using Machine (Nautilus Freedom Trainer pictured)

Keep your abdominals tight and your weight on your heels, not your toes. Do not allow your thighs to go past parallel on the squat (although on a leg press machine you can go deeper as comfort allows). Do not bounce to get back up. Do 12 to 15 reps. If you are unable to perform squats or leg presses because of patellar issues, see Patellar Pain Syndrome on page 159 and consider the Horse, Partial Wall Seat, Quad Isometrics, or "Short Arcs" on pages 74, 123, 154, and 155 instead of this exercise.

2. With Tubing

3. With Free Weights

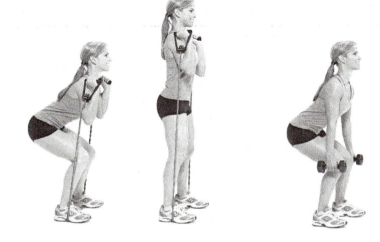

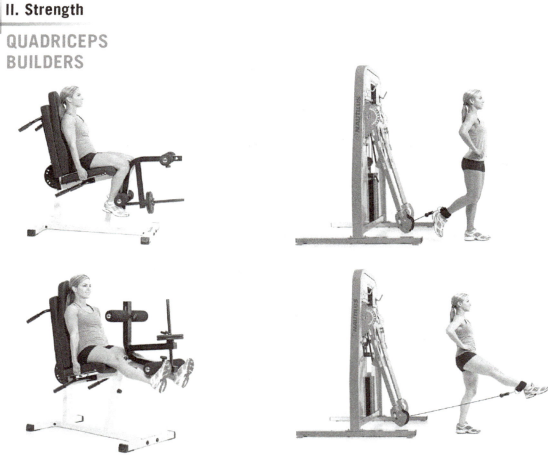

Leg Extensions (3 variations)

1. Seated on Machine

Perform the lift slowly, concentrating on tightening the quadriceps at the end of the movement. If you have patellar problems, omit this exercise and follow the suggestions on Patellar Pain Syndrome on page 159. Often patellar problems are in a midrange of the exercise, so you can work the muscle in your partial comfort range. This includes pinning the weight stack out so that you are electing only the last 15 to 20 degrees of extension. This "short arc" version can be done either on a machine or even with ankle weights (see concentration VMO "Short Arc" on page 155). Also, seat adjustment is important in avoiding patellar issues. Too far forward or backward puts undue pressure on the kneecap.

2. Using Nautilus Freedom Trainer (or equivalent)

This exercise can also be performed using elastic tubing and a door attachment.

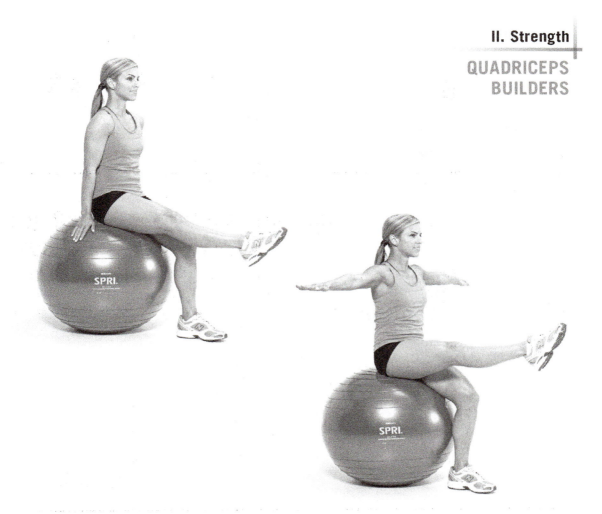

3. Seated on Ball

This exercise will improve your balance as well as your core, quadriceps, and hamstring strength. Sit on the ball, tall and upright, with your feet no more than shoulder-width apart and your hands resting on the sides of the ball. Tighten your abdominal muscles. Keeping one foot flat on the floor, extend your other leg fully, tightening your thigh muscles. Hold for 10 seconds. Repeat 5 times with each leg. If your hamstrings are tight, you will not be able to fully straighten your leg, but go to where it is comfortable and hold that position, trying to improve each time.

Advanced version:

Remove your hands from the ball and keep them out to the sides so your body forms a T. For even more of a challenge, add ankle weights, starting with 1 or 2 pounds. Also try doing this while on the ball of your foot, rather than keeping your foot flat on the floor.

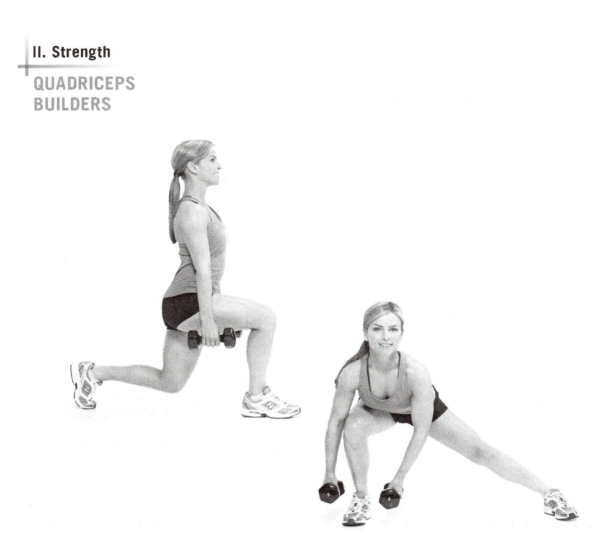

Lunges

Start with both feet together, with or without weights. Slowly lunge forward so that your thigh is parallel to the ground and your knee remains directly over your foot. Hold for 2 to 3 seconds before rising back up. Do 10 reps on each side. Add weights as you get stronger. Alternatives include the side lunge (above) or walking lunges (in which you walk forward or backward into the lunge position).

HAMSTRING BUILDERS

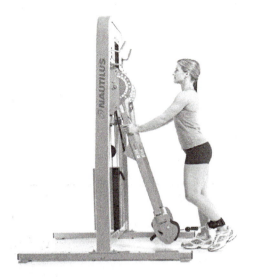

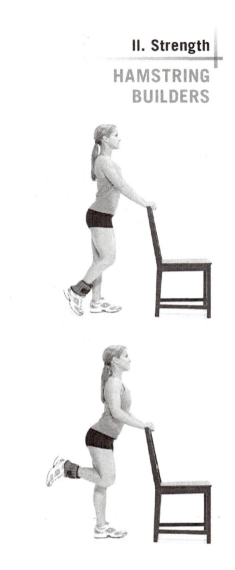

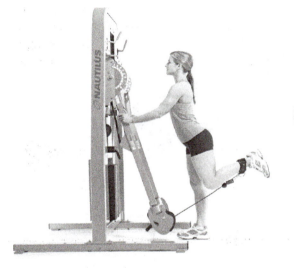

Leg Curl with Nautilus Freedom Trainer (or equivalent)

Do not arch your back as you bring your foot toward your buttocks. Do not raise the weight rapidly. Let the weight back down slowly in a controlled manner. Do 10 repetitions and repeat using the opposite leg.

Alternates: Try a standing kickback with tubing or ankle weights, or standing leg curls with ankle weights.

HAMSTRING BUILDERS

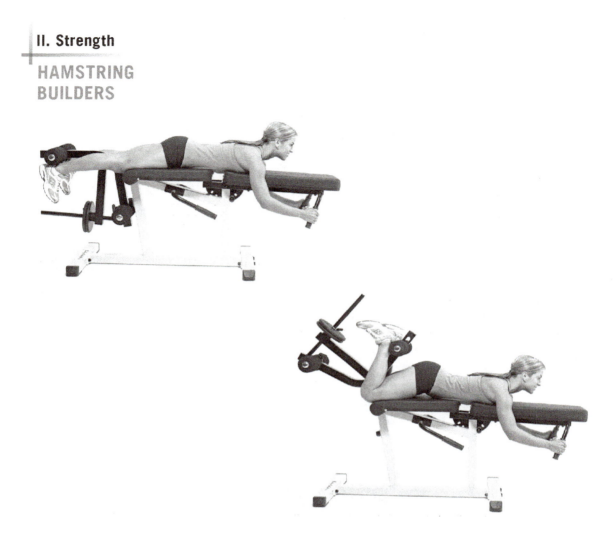

Leg Curl on Machine

Lie facedown and slowly flex both legs so that your heels come toward your buttocks. Pause for 1 or 2 seconds, then slowly lower your legs to the starting position. Try not to arch your back (especially if you have lower back issues), and do not look upward if you have neck problems. This exercise can also be done using one leg at a time. Do 10 to 12 reps.

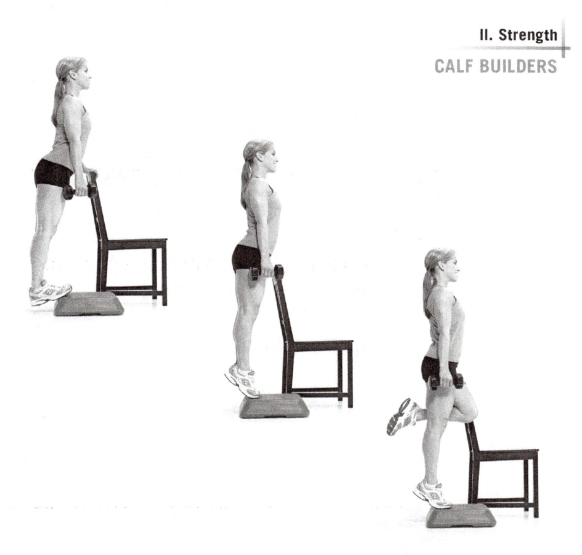

Calf Raises

Problems with residual calf weakness (both strength and endurance) follow many lower-extremity injuries, from the foot up to the hip. This exercise can be done using both legs at once or one at a time. (With machines, I prefer both legs at once; when working off a step or on flat ground, I prefer one leg at a time.) If you can do 20 calf raises on each side without weights, then start adding weights to either the machine or by holding dumbbells in your hands.

HIPS AND PELVIS

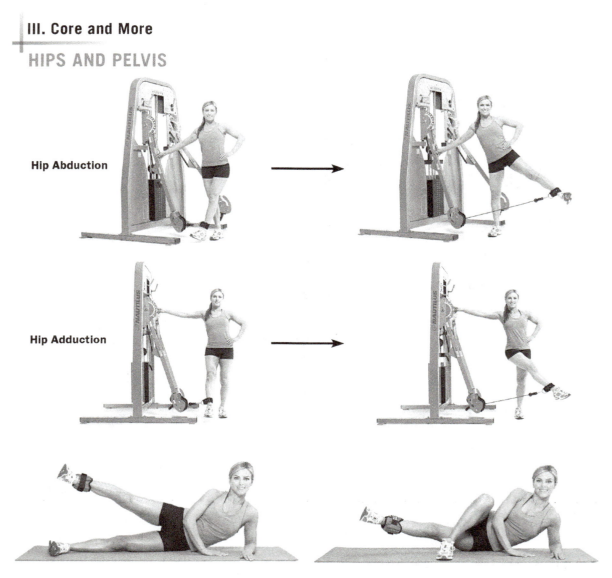

Hip Abduction

Hip Adduction

Abductor and Adductor

These can be done with a machine, ankle weights, or tubing. Move your leg slowly in a controlled manner. Do not bounce, especially when your legs are wide apart and are being pulled back inward. Your movements should be controlled. Do not lean. If you have restricted hip movement, stay within your pain-free range of motion. Tighten your abs during the movement. Do 10 to 12 reps on each side.

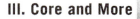

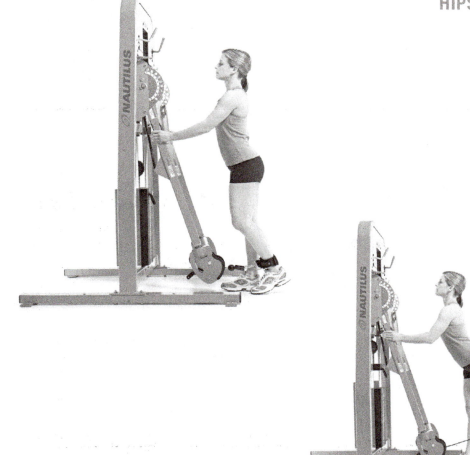

Kickback (Hamstrings and Gluteals)

Do not arch your back. While holding on for support, lift your leg
against resistance (weights or tubing) in a slow, controlled manner.
Do 10 to 12 reps and repeat with your opposite leg.

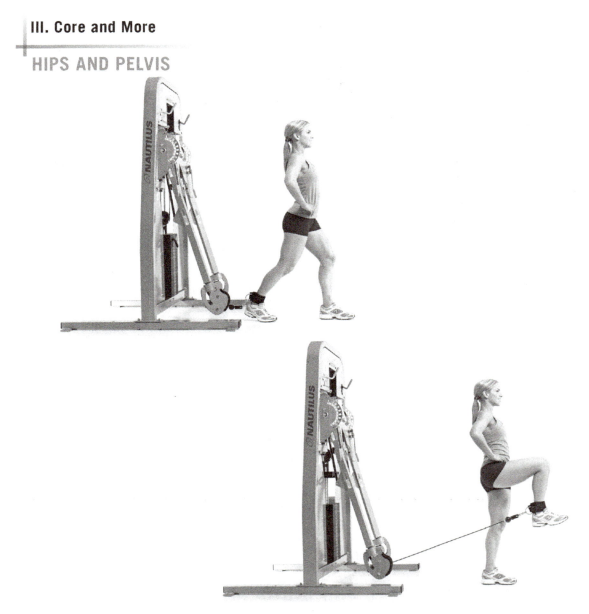

Forward Flexion (Hip Flexors)

Slowly lift your knee upward and forward so your thigh is parallel to the ground. Hold for 2 seconds and let down. Do 10 to 12 reps and repeat with the opposite leg.

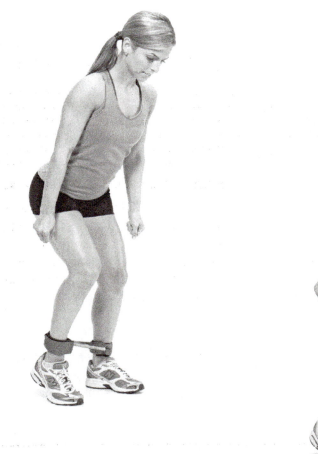
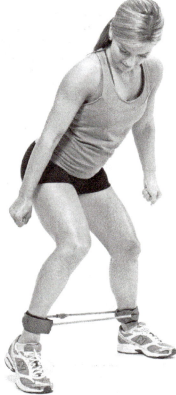

Side Walk with Tubing

Wrap elastic tubing around your ankle area so that it is under mild tension. Flex your knees slightly and slowly take large steps to the side. Try 10 steps in each direction. Also try walking in diagonal patterns, forward and backward. Tighten the tension on the tubing as your strength and endurance improve.

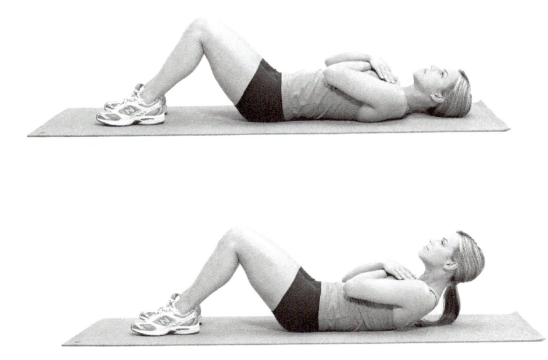

Crunch

Lie on the floor with your knees bent and feet flat. Start with a pelvic tilt maneuver, tightening your abs and partially flattening your lower back toward the floor. Do not throw yourself forward. Do not clasp your hands behind your head, but keep them near your ears or across your chest. Do not anchor your feet under anything or have someone hold your feet, as this allows you to use your hip flexor muscles rather than your abs.

Tighten your abdominal muscles and slowly curl your head and shoulders off the floor; feel your breastbone accordion in toward your upper pubic bone. Don't come up past 30 degrees as you would in an old-fashioned situp. Don't use your hands to pull your neck or head forward, and keep your lower back on the floor. Pause momentarily; then, very slowly, in a controlled manner, come back down. Slowly exhale during the lifting phase and inhale during the lowering

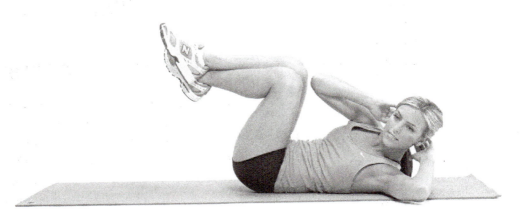

phase. You should feel the movement, the "burn," in your abs. Concentrate on the feeling in your abs, and not how high you can lift off. Do 20 reps (add more each day as you get better).

Note: In most gyms, there are great machine options for total abdominal work, and they include the ab machines or machine crunch as well as the rotary torso for obliques. There are also numerous alternatives that are worth incorporating into your workouts at various times. The basic crunch tends to work the upper abdominal area. To target your lower abdominal area, do a hanging knee raise from a chinup bar or do a reverse crunch in which you keep your head and shoulders on the ground and slowly bring your knees upward and then downward.

Advanced version—Crunch with a Twist

Lie on your back with your ankles crossed and your hips and knees flexed at 90-degree angles. Slowly perform a crunch, bringing your right elbow to your left knee. Hold for 3 seconds. Do 10 repetitions and repeat on the opposite side. (For a slightly easier version, lie on your back with your right knee bent and foot resting on the floor. Cross your left leg over your right knee, keeping your left arm out on the floor. Place your right hand near your right ear and slowly twist up, bringing your right elbow toward your left knee.)

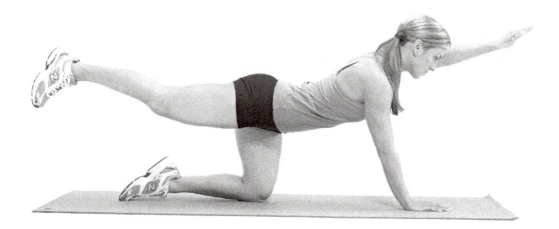

Bird Dog

Start on the floor on all fours. Slowly lift your left arm and right leg simultaneously, holding both straight for 5 to 7 seconds. Do not raise your arm or leg above horizontal; instead, stay parallel to the floor. Alternate sides and do 5 reps on each side.

Modified version: If the full Bird Dog is too difficult, or if you have significant discomfort, try raising only one arm or one leg at a time, and gradually build up to where you can hold both out, even if they are only partially held out rather than fully.

Advanced version: Using ankle weights and a small hand weight, add 3 to 5 pounds per limb.

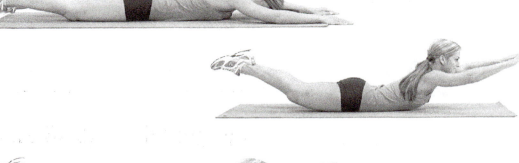

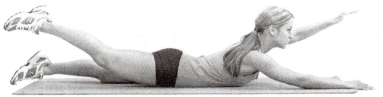

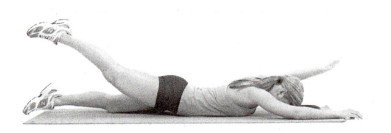

Superman

I first described this exercise almost 30 years ago both to assess spinal strength and to help individuals rebuild their lower backs after injury. This exercise is terrific for spinal extensor muscle strength and maintaining overall spine health.

Lie on the floor facedown with your arms straight out, in line with your legs. (Picture Superman flying in the air.) Simultaneously bring both arms and both legs off the floor. Only your abdominal area and pelvis should be touching the floor. Hold for 10 seconds and build up to 20 seconds. Do 10 reps.

Modified version: If the above is too difficult or causes too much discomfort, raise your left arm and right leg off the floor. Keep your knee straight so that your leg is being lifted by your buttocks and lower back. If it does not bother your neck, your head should also come off the floor. Hold for 10 seconds and build up to 20 seconds. Repeat with your right arm and left leg. Do 3 reps on each side. (If you have neck problems, you can keep your face resting on the floor and not lift your head.) If you are unable to do even this version, you can start with just lifting only one arm or leg off the floor and build up as tolerated.

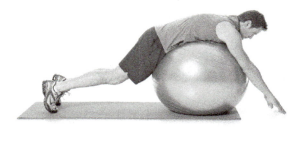

Superman on Ball

This exercise is for spinal extensor and gluteal muscle strength and endurance.

Lie facedown on the ball with your toes touching the floor and your arms stretched out in front, reaching forward. Let your spine and entire body relax. Hold for 20 to 30 seconds or as long as you like if you find this comfortable. This is a good lower back stretch and relaxation exercise and is good to do before starting the actual Superman movement.

Keeping your feet on the floor and your legs straight, slowly extend your lumbar area until you are straight or slightly extended in the lower back area and your arms are fully extended beyond your head, like Superman flying. Hold for 10 seconds and build up to 20 seconds. Do 5 to 10 reps.

More advanced version: Get into the Superman position and then gently lift one straight leg off the floor, balancing only on the opposite straightened leg. Hold for 5 seconds, then alternate legs.

Most advanced version: Do the full Superman, in which only your abdominal area is on the ball and both feet and arms are outward in the "flying" position. Feet should be off the floor.

Modified version: If you are unable to perform the above, start by assisting yourself, keeping your hands on the floor and just slightly lifting them off the floor when possible. Gradually build up to where you can straighten your back fully and then start bringing your hands upward to the full Superman.

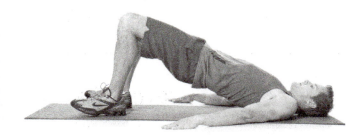

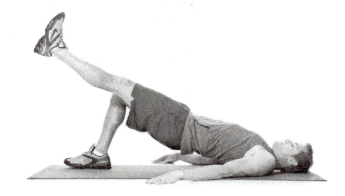

Glute Bridge (with leg up)

Lie on the floor with your knees bent to 90 degrees, your feet flat on the floor and hip-width apart, and your arms away from your body (at 45-degree angles) and resting on the floor to support you. Tighten your abs and lift or bridge your hips toward the ceiling while tightening your glutes (buttock muscles). Next, slowly extend your left leg so that it is straight out, toes pointing toward the ceiling. Hold your left leg out for 5 seconds and then lower it, maintaining the firm bridge position at all times throughout this exercise until all reps are completed. Repeat with your right leg. Complete 10 reps with each leg.

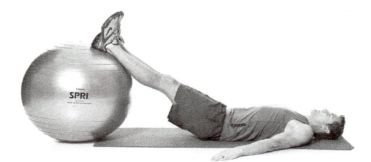

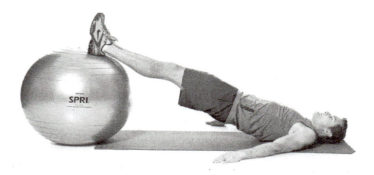

Glute Bridge on Ball

Lie on the floor with your heels on the ball and toes pointing upward, arms and palms resting flat on the floor slightly away from your body. Tighten your glutes, lifting your pelvis upward to form a straight line. Only your head, shoulders, and arms will be on the floor. Hold for 3 seconds and slowly drop back down to the floor. Repeat 5 times.

Advanced version: Try crossing your arms in front of your chest, making balance more difficult.

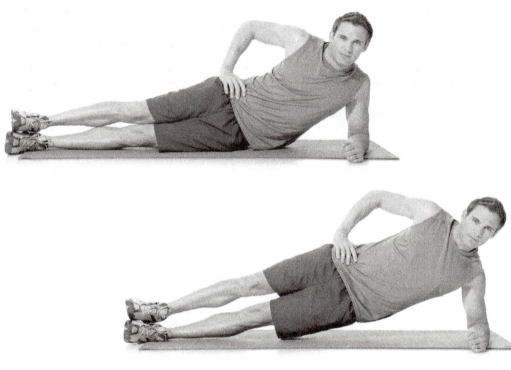

Side Plank on Floor

Lie on your left side, with your left forearm and elbow on the floor. Your elbow should be in line with your shoulder, and your torso sagging toward the floor. Lean on your forearm, lifting your hips and knees upward into a straight, rigid line while supporting all your weight on your forearm and the side of your left foot. Hold for 20 seconds. Repeat twice and then perform the exercise again, lying on your right side.

Alternate version:
Instead of stacking one foot directly on the other, try performing this plank with the foot of the top leg also resting on the floor just in front of your other foot.

Advanced version: Try to increase your hold time to 1 to 2 minutes. If this gets too easy, hold a light weight against the hip that's on top.

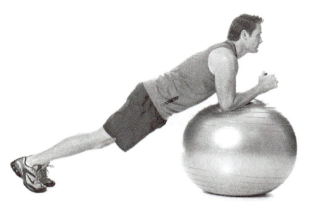

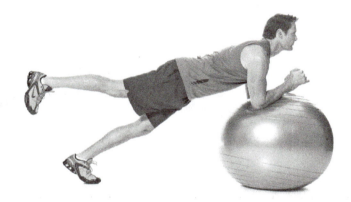

Bridge/Plank on Ball

Kneel facing a ball, resting your elbows and forearms on the ball. Tighten your abs and lift upward into the Plank position so that your back and legs form a straight line and you are supported only on your elbows and feet. Hold for 20 seconds, keeping your abs and torso area tightened and stabilized. Repeat twice. Try to build up to 1 minute.

Advanced version: Once you are stabilized and secure, slowly lift your right leg in a straight line using your gluteal muscles. Hold for 20 seconds and then change legs. Repeat twice with each leg.

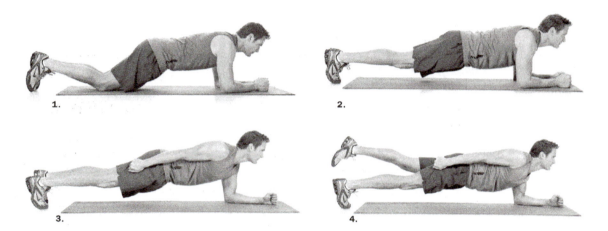

1.
2.
3.
4.

Quadruped

While kneeling on the floor, place your forearms flat on the floor as if you were to do a modi-fied pushup. Now, assume the plank position with your body straight and your full weight supported on both forearms and your toes (second photo). Your body should be straight as a board with your pelvis tucked inward, tightening your abdominal muscles. Try holding that position with your weight on your forearms and toes for 60 seconds.

Next, lift your right arm off the floor for 15 seconds, supporting your full weight on your left arm and both feet (third photo). Repeat, lifting your left arm.

With both forearms on the floor, raise your right leg, hold for 15 seconds, and then repeat, lifting your left leg.

Next, try to elevate your right arm and left leg simultaneously (fourth photo) and hold for 15 seconds, then return them to the floor and repeat with your left arm and right leg raised.

Return to the plank position and hold for 30 seconds.

IV. Neuromuscular Training

The first two exercises below can help anyone. The other three are primarily for athletes and very active individuals who strive to perform at an advanced level. (For additional neuromuscular training information, see the section on ACL injuries on page 22 and Additional Resources on page 194.)

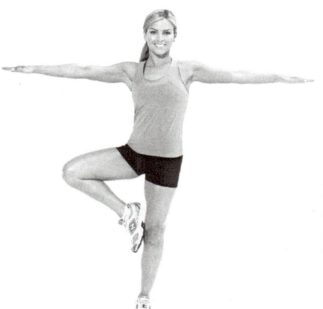

The Stork

Stand up straight, extend your arms out wide to your sides, then raise one foot off the ground to the level of the opposite knee. Rest the arch of your foot on the inner side of your knee, forming the letter P. Try not to sway or rock to maintain balance. Hold for 10 seconds on each foot; try to build up to 20 seconds. (This is a good time to practice your relaxation breathing as you exercise.)

Advanced version: As this gets easier, try to perform it with your eyes closed, on the ball of your foot, or on a small firm pillow (or a wobble board or Bosu trainer if available).

Note: This is a simple way to improve your balance, and it will help with injury and fall prevention as well as improving sports performance. If you have had an injury (especially knee, foot, or ankle), this may be difficult, but it is an important part of your total recovery. If you have difficulty with this exercise, you should perform it several times per day, every day.

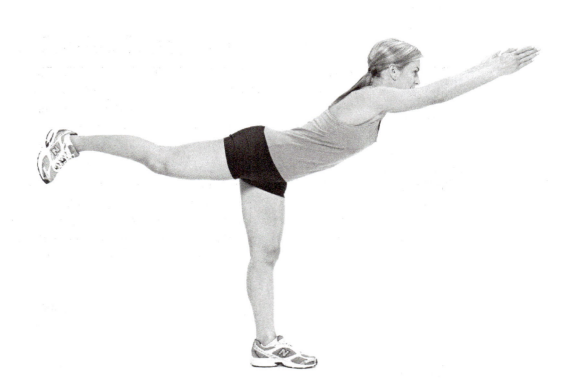

The Warrior

Looking straight ahead, balance on your left leg while slowly lifting your right leg backward and extending your arms and hands forward. Bend forward until you feel a stretch in the hamstrings of your left leg. Balance on the left leg forming a T with the rest of your body. Keep your back flat and avoid twisting. Hold for 20 to 30 seconds while breathing comfortably. Repeat, starting on your right leg.

Advanced version: As this gets easier, try to perform it with your eyes closed.

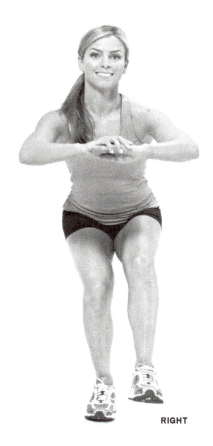

RIGHT

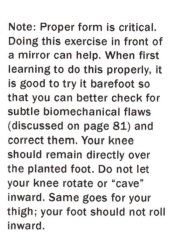

WRONG

Single-Leg Squat

This improves leg strength, dynamic flexibility, and neuromuscular control.

Stand upright with your left foot raised. Slowly lower your body so your knee is bent approximately 45 degrees; keep your back straight. Do 10 to 15 reps and repeat on the opposite side. (If this becomes too easy, you can add resistance by holding dumbbells in both hands, or even try it on an uneven surface like a Bosu trainer or half foam roll.)

Note: Proper form is critical. Doing this exercise in front of a mirror can help. When first learning to do this properly, it is good to try it barefoot so that you can better check for subtle biomechanical flaws (discussed on page 81) and correct them. Your knee should remain directly over the planted foot. Do not let your knee rotate or "cave" inward. Same goes for your thigh; your foot should not roll inward.

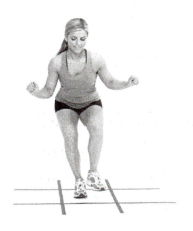

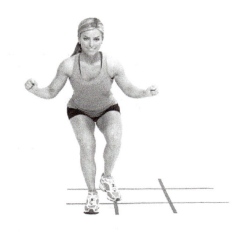

Tic-Tac-Toe Bunny Hop

Use duct tape or masking tape to make a large tic-tac-toe grid on the floor (so that both feet comfortably fit in each square). Stand in the center square on one foot. Bunny hop one square at a time forward and backward. Next try side to side, followed by diagonal patterns. Start with 30 seconds on each leg and build up to 60 seconds.

Your right and left leg should perform equally (this is not often the case if there have been knee problems, injury, or surgery). Landings should be soft and controlled and not a "thud." The knee should point straight ahead and be directly over your foot without the tendency to buckle inward or shake.

Advanced version:
When the drill on the tic-tac-toe grid becomes too easy, you can advance to hopping over small rubber cones. Include double-leg lateral hops as well as double-leg forward/backward hops. Progress to single-leg hopping over cones. Always be sure that your form is perfect and does not deteriorate with repetitive hops before moving to the next advanced level.

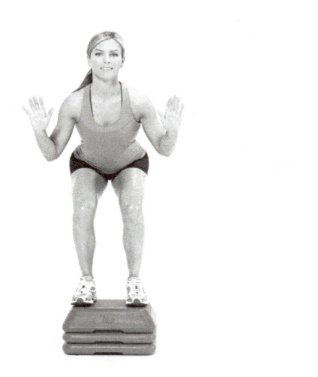

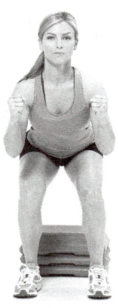

CORRECT LANDING

Drop Jump

Note: Before trying this, see the caution on the opposite page.

Stand on a solid box or platform approximately 12 inches high (the bottom one or two steps of a staircase or the stackable steps found in aerobic studios can work as well). Jump off and land simultaneously onto both feet (pointing forward and parallel—picture a gymnast "sticking" the landing). As you get better at this, you can increase the height of the step or platform, and also try jumping higher or onto one leg.

Strive for a soft but solid square landing with your knees bent and directly over your feet. Practice in front of a mirror or have someone videotape you. Those prone to knee injury will land with the knee straight (and/or hyperextended) or they will land flexed, but the knees will buckle inward (toward each other) ever so slightly. Try a few times in a row to see if you fatigue easily or if your form begins to suffer. Also, before trying this on a higher box, platform, or step, you may want to try on level ground or a small step.

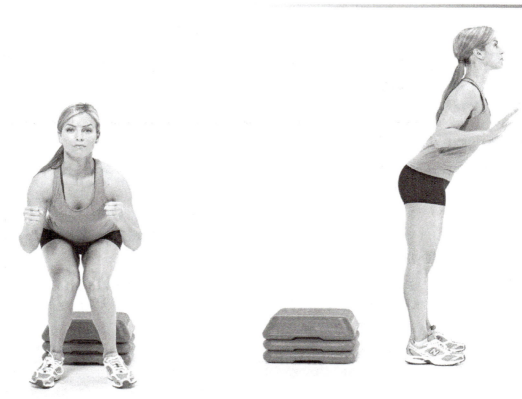

IMPROPER LANDING

CAUTION: You probably should hold off on this if any of the following apply to you:

❏ You're not athletic and not used to jumping.

❏ You don't do sports and don't plan to.

❏ Your knee is painful or swollen and/or you have instability issues.

❏ You have knee weakness and/or had a recent injury or surgery.

❏ You have balance or fall issues.

In the above cases, a doctor or physical therapist can assess when the time is right for this important knee parameter.

RECOVERY AND INJURY-SPECIFIC REHAB AND EXERCISE PROGRAMS

While wind sprints can be great training for an athlete, one mad dash can lead to hospitalization, or even death, for someone with a heart problem.

Almost everyone seems to accept that distinction, but somehow the same cautionary logic hasn't extended to the musculoskeletal system, including the knee region. Some muscle-building and exercise routines, while great for healthy young knees, are dangerous for others. There may be nothing wrong with the exercises themselves; they just aren't right for certain knee conditions. And there may be other exercises that can resolve or at least improve the problem.

A vital part of the FrameWork program is a collection of exercises modified for certain ailments. This slight adjustment in approach—The FrameWork Fix—not only makes the movements safe, but also contributes to repair and recovery. So there is no excuse for hanging up your workout duds if you have a weak or injured knee. (All the more reason to lace up those sneaks, in fact.)

Just be sure to incorporate the appropriate modifications.

It bears repeating that if you are under the care of a physician or therapist, you must run the following program by him or her for approval, especially if you've had a recent surgery.

Recovery

Recovery exercises are simple, low stress, and yet highly effective exercises for individuals who are in the early recovery phase from an injury, surgery, or anything that has the knee down and out. It could even be arthritis or some other type of flare-up; the knee is often swollen to some extent, still painful, and probably a little stiff. You may be limping and even still using crutches, a cane, or a walker, but you have been given the go-ahead by your physician to start moving and regaining strength, motion, and function. When the knee is a little swollen or sore, muscle atrophy occurs pretty rapidly and further stiffness could set in.

These exercises will help prevent that. Also, if you are able to exercise your healthy leg in the usual manner, that can actually help prevent atrophy in the injured or painful side. This is another reason that we in sports medicine try to keep all of the healthy frame parts active and moving while the injured ones heal.

JOINT DISCUSSION

Neuromuscular training has come front and center in the world of sports performance and injury prevention. There are numerous techniques, including plyometrics and other agility drills, designed for this purpose, and the programs continue to evolve with more and more scientific evidence supporting their use. In this book, we introduce some sample routines but also urge you to do more research and talk to your orthopedic surgeon, physical therapist, and athletic trainer to point you in the right direction for more specific individualized instruction. All young athletes, especially females, should be involved in these preventive training programs. Parents and coaches must take a more proactive stance in this regard, and I remain baffled as to why neuromuscular training is not being offered routinely in schools and on playing fields across the country.

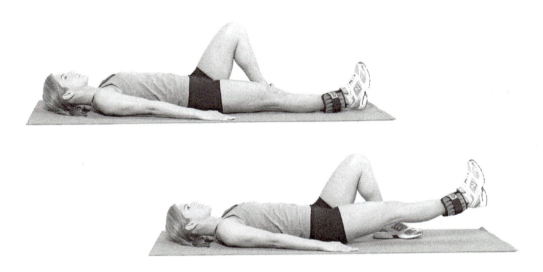

Lock-and-Lift Isometrics

This exercise is ideal for anyone in the early phases of knee rehabilitation, especially post-op, including arthroscopy. All too often I see motivated individuals trying to strengthen their quad muscles when their "cheatin' bod" is playing tricks. This is especially true when you are doing quad isometrics, or straight leg lifts, when your body is wrongly using your hip flexors, not your quadriceps and particularly not your important VMO (vastus medialis obliquus) portion of the quad—a teardrop-shaped muscle on the inner side of the knee just above the kneecap— to raise the leg. To avoid this, I developed the concentration "lock-and-lift" exercise.

Lie on your back with your left knee bent and left foot resting on the floor. Next, tighten and slowly lock your right thigh (pushing back with the right knee). Feel the VMO muscle; be sure it contracts and gets firm. Next, lift your right leg 6 to 8 inches off the floor and hold 5 to 7 seconds. Keep feeling your thigh muscle and VMO to be sure they are staying tight at maximal contraction (until you get really good at this). Hold for 5 to 7 seconds and repeat 12 to 15 times. When this gets very easy, start adding ankle weights; begin with 1 to 2 pounds and don't go over 10 pounds, or you will probably start using your hip again to do the lift. The key is concentrating on tightening and palpating the muscle for biofeedback-type information to assure you are really working the muscle effectively. Next, perform this exercise on the opposite leg, if needed.

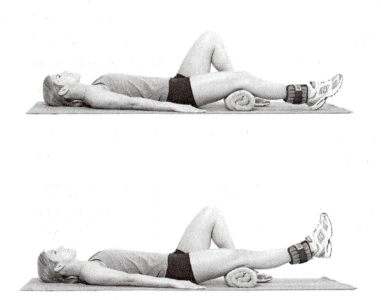

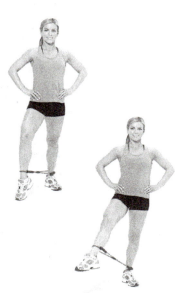

Concentration VMO "Short Arc"

Lie on the floor with your left knee flexed and your left foot flat on the floor. Your right leg should have a rolled towel under the knee. Using your quad (front thigh) muscle, lift your right heel off the ground, tightening the thigh until your right leg is fully straightened. (Do not use the front of your hip to lift the leg off the towel. You should be pressing back slightly with your right knee to squeeze and flatten the towel.) Feel your VMO to make sure it is tight and stays tight for the 5 to 7 seconds you hold the leg straight. Repeat with the other leg.

Alternate version— T-Band Pumps: Tie elastic tubing or a Theraband around your ankles with your feet approximately shoulder-width apart. Turn the affected leg outward slightly (as shown in the photo), allowing the knee to flex slightly. Lift the foot off the ground and perform a pumping-action, thigh-tightening, knee-straightening exercise with the elastic as resistance. Do 3 sets of 20 reps. Repeat with the other leg if needed.

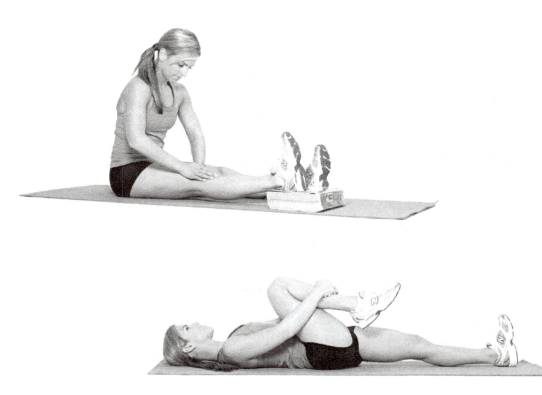

Knee Range-of-Motion

Place your heel on a phone book and gently press downward on your knee until it is fully extended. Hold for 5 seconds. Next, flex your knee and gently pull your heel toward your buttocks, holding for the same count. Try to improve your motion a little more in each session. This can be done multiple times per day, especially if your knee is stiff. This exercise accomplishes two things: It can help regain lost motion and mobility, and it can help prevent further motion loss even if you don't regain full motion.

INJURY-SPECIFIC REHAB AND EXERCISE PROGRAMS

Share my world a bit—there is a Top 10 list of the most common ailments and injuries I see day in and day out (the "Recovery" knee listed above and the nine listed below). They're the ones *FrameWork for the Knee* aims to prevent, improve, or even resolve. (For more information about these conditions, see the Sports Medicine section of my Web site, www.drnick .com, or the patient education area of the American Academy of Orthopaedic Surgeons (AAOS) Web site, "Your Orthopaedic Connection," at www.orthoinfo.aaos.org.)

The exercise modifications and additions that follow a brief review of each injury should be included in your workout and/or rehabilitation. Remember, rehab-type exercises can and should be done daily, even several times a day, until normal strength and/or flexibility are regained and you're feeling good. You often need several sets, especially a warmup with lighter weights or resistance for the strength exercises.

It's even more important to listen to your body, monitoring yourself for any significant discomfort or other changes to suggest you are getting further into trouble rather than out of it. This is especially true as you start to resume more normal workouts, although I recommend always giving your weak links a little added attention. As you expand your routine, especially as it involves the problem area or areas, don't add more than one new exercise per workout. While you're at the gym, you often feel great, only to be sore or even in pain that evening or the following day. When you add more than one exercise, it's hard to know which is the culprit and needs either further modification or exclusion. This is another instance when some detective work is in order. And again, remember: If you're under the care of a physician or other health-care professional, always check with him or her about any changes in your program.

Knee Arthritis

As we have said before, the incidence of knee arthritis is sharply on the rise, and arthritis is the number-one cause of activity limitation in adults in our nation. Unfortunately, we are also seeing it in younger and younger patients. Pain, stiffness, and weakness are all common, and patients often find themselves in a downward spiral and the vicious cycle we mentioned in Step 2. It is essential to break that cycle, and exercise is one of the keys—but it must be done in a way that doesn't overly irritate the knee.

Temporary, relatively mild discomfort is to be expected, and if you can work through that, you will improve. No two knees are alike when it comes to arthritis, and what works for someone else may not work for you. Also, depending on the location of the arthritis within your knee (i.e., patella versus medial and/or lateral compartment or a combination of these), some activities and exercises are better tolerated, and some will precipitate a flare-up. So you need to monitor your progress and be prepared to make some adjustments.

The Framework Fix: Eliminate high-impact exercises like running. Instead, try a bicycle, an elliptical machine, or water-based exercises. If you are able to walk, that's fine; gradually try to build up your time. I prefer a good running sneaker over a walking sneaker because the better cushioning means less stress to your knees. The goal is to build up to 30 minutes a day of any of these aerobic-type exercises. If a full 30 minutes is not possible, try three 10-minute sessions spread over the day. It all adds up to a healthier you.

For strengthening, do Lock-and-Lift Isometrics (page 154); if tolerated, move up to "Short Arcs" (page 155), then to leg extensions (page 126). Add quad and hamstring stretching (pages 113 and 114). Do Knee Range-of-Motion exercises (page 156) to gain or maintain mobility. Also do calf strengthening (page 131).

Knee Cartilage or Meniscus Tear

This extremely common injury is to baseball catchers what turned ankles are to basketball players. Football players tear cartilage when they get clipped or do a sudden twist. Weight lifters tear theirs by using poor form or deep squats—bouncing in sudden exertion when trying to lift too much weight. Plumbers, auto mechanics, and other "squatters" can get a rip just doing their jobs. So can mothers helping their kids "button up."

The menisci—those C-shaped shock absorbers in each knee—simply dry out and weaken with age. When that happens, you can tear your cartilage just getting out of a car or working in your garden. Then you need arthroscopic surgery, which isn't so bad, but in removing the damaged cartilage, you are also removing a shock absorber. So that gives you another weak link.

Stronger surrounding muscles can compensate to some extent. To protect your knees, give that surrounding tissue a good workout. Meanwhile, be mindful of other ways to both lower the stresses on your knees and improve the shock absorption.

The FrameWork Fix: Do stationary bicycling, which is great to build both quad strength and endurance to help with knee shock absorption. Do quad strengthening (page 122), Knee Range-of-Motion exercises (page 156), calf and hamstring strengthening (pages 131 and 133), hip and core strengthening (page 132), and neuromuscular training (page 146).

If you have had a meniscal repair whereby it was actually stitched and saved, you will have more restrictions in terms of what is allowed in the early post-op phase. Talk to your surgeon about what you can and can't do. For example, because meniscal repairs are slow to heal, running is often not allowed for 12 to 16 weeks after surgery, depending on the size and location of the tear. For those who have had a meniscal allograft (donor replacement of the meniscus), the post-op program is even more strict and is best outlined by your surgeon. Once you are given the green light to exercise, incorporate those listed above.

Patellar Pain Syndrome

An irritated patella (kneecap) is the number-one knee problem among younger people. During adolescence, growth spurts in bones sometimes mean that muscle and tendons can't keep up, which leaves kids with dangerously tight hamstrings. Malalignment can mean that the kneecap doesn't ride properly in its groove. In adults, the same condition is created by overuse and imbalance (as in too much running without adequate stretching and strengthening exercises to offset the self-imposed imbalances and tightness) as well as wear and tear.

With age and with injuries, simple wear and tear can lead to degenerative arthritis under the kneecap. Most exercises that strengthen the thigh will irritate this already troubled spot, so you have to be very smart and strategic in your workouts. In this context, step aerobics, squats, and leg extensions are all "X-rated," meaning that you don't go there. Quadriceps strengthening is the answer, but it has to be done so as not to overload the kneecap. Hamstring and iliotibial band (ITB) stretching are also essential.

The FrameWork Fix: Eliminate quad exercises (leg extensions, lunges, squats). Add Lock-and-Lift Isometrics (page 154) or "lock out" or "pin out" the weight stack on machines to minimize arc. If this starting point is tolerated, then add "Short Arc" isotonics and T-Band Pumps (page 155). Stretch quads, hamstrings, and the ITB (pages 113, 114, and 118). Also strengthen hip adductors (most important) and hip abductors (page 132) as well as your core and pelvic area. Add stationary bicycling but with a higher seat position, no hills, and use toe clips, or use the elliptical machine. Avoid stair-steppers, especially many of the inexpensive home versions that might not be as smooth for your knee. If you must use a stepper, keep the step action on one of the lower settings. Consider a knee sleeve (neoprene with an opening for the patella).

Infrapatellar Tendinitis

This is an all-too-common complaint among basketball and volleyball players, as well as dancers, so much so that they often think it's normal to get a "pinch" of pain when they jump or land. Runners feel it, too, especially on a downhill slope. Usually, a tight, overdeveloped quadriceps muscle is putting a strain on the tendon that lives just below the kneecap. The answer is quad stretching, as well as exercises that emphasize the eccentric or lengthening contraction on the muscle, the one we experience when we properly (i.e., slowly) lower a weight.

The FrameWork Fix: Add transverse friction massage (direct pressure on the sore tendon area, fingers across fibers), quad, hamstring, and calf stretching (pages 113, 114, and 121), and the Eccentric Quad Strengthening exercise on the opposite page. Consider a "Cho-Pat" strap (a band that goes around the knee just below the tip of the kneecap) or a knee sleeve.

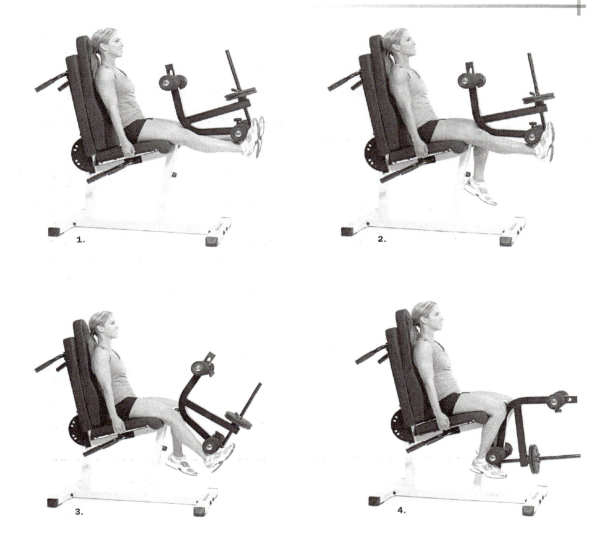

1.
2.
3.
4.

Eccentric Quad Strengthening

Do double leg extensions, then slowly relax the uninvolved leg down and lower the weight with the involved side only. This allows for negative, or eccentric, quad work.

ITB Friction Syndrome

Repetitive movement of this thick, tendonlike structure on the outer side of the knee can create friction bursitis. Cyclists and runners get this frequently, and technical factors play a big role. For cyclists, it's not just the height of the seat that matters but its place forward or aft. The problem for runners is often banked surfaces or legs that are uneven in length.

The FrameWork Fix: Try the Pretzel ITB stretch (page 118), T-Roll (page 116), Piriformis stretch (page 120), and the Wall Stretch (opposite) and Toe Touch with Legs Crossed (page 164). Do core work as well as gluteal and hip abductor and adductor strengthening with elastic (pages 132 to 135). Consider orthotics. Check knee alignment (page 73) and leg-length discrepancy (if one leg is longer than the other). If you are a runner or walker, avoid banked surfaces. If you bike, check your seat adjustment (up/down and front/back), and use toe clips.

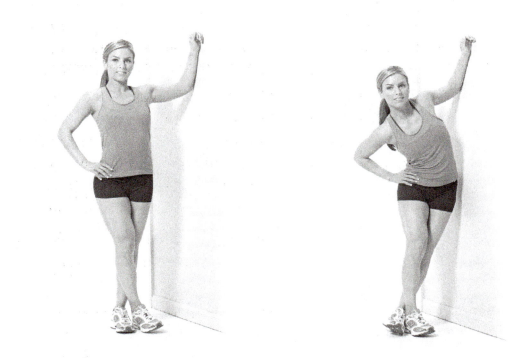

Wall Stretch

Stand about 1 foot from a wall. To stretch your left outer hip and ITB, cross your left leg behind your right one and rest your extended elbow out to the wall for support. Next, let your left hip sag toward the wall as shown. Hold for 20 seconds and repeat 3 times. Do the same for the opposite side. As you gain flexibility, you can move slightly out farther from the wall.

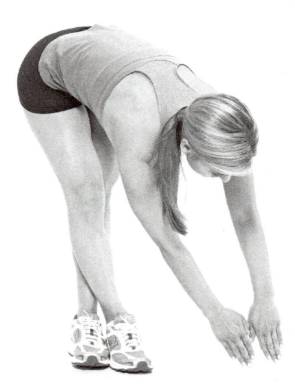

Toe Touch with Legs Crossed

To stretch your right ITB, cross your legs in front of you, with your right leg in the forward position (this will stretch your right ITB). Flex forward and lean toward your left side. Hold for 20 seconds and repeat 3 times. You should feel a stretch in your outer right hip and thigh area. Repeat with the opposite side if needed.

ACL Tear (Trick Knee)

The anterior cruciate ligament is a ropelike band of tissue that runs through the center of the knee and helps to hold the joint together. When it tears, the shin bone (tibia) can slide forward in relation to the thigh bone (femur). That's the "trick" in a trick knee, an excruciatingly painful stunt you'll never want to repeat.

Surgery can repair most of the damage, but prevention—strengthening the core, hip, hamstrings, and quads, and improving proprioception, agility, and balance the way dancers do—is vastly preferable. We are now learning that many ACL tears are preventable with certain year-round conditioning programs, especially those that focus on strengthening and functional drills that include jumping and landing routines. These programs are especially important for young female athletes, who are tearing their ACLs at epidemic rates. I believe that every young athlete, especially females, should be on an ACL preventive program as part of their routine practices and training on and off the field. Programs like the Santa Monica ACL Prevention Project (www.aclprevent.com) mentioned earlier are excellent.

The FrameWork Fix: Take a lesson from dancers, who, unlike most female athletes, rarely ever tear their ACLs. In addition to the exercises below, do comprehensive leg and knee strengthening, especially hamstrings. Backward walking on a treadmill helps to build and strengthen hamstrings. Core strength is also protective. Add tai chi and dance moves as well as the neuromuscular training exercises beginning on page 146.

If you have had ACL surgery, especially in the first 6 months post-op, you should follow your surgeon's guidelines for recovery. I believe in a fairly aggressive rehab program starting almost immediately post-op, but every surgeon is different depending on his or her philosophy, the type of graft and techniques used, and the method of graft fixation in the knee. If you are more than 6 months out of surgery, or if you are trying to live without an ACL (i.e., the ligament tore and you never had surgery), then the following routines will be helpful.

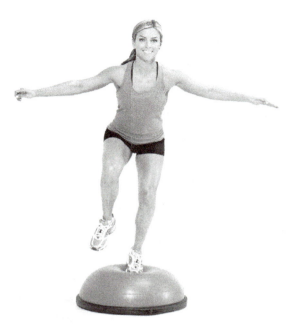

BALANCE TRAINING

A wobble board or Bosu trainer is a small platform that supports a half ball. By practicing balancing and standing on this inherently unstable object, you can significantly improve your proprioception.

FOUR-QUADRANT HOPPING DRILLS

After you are able to comfortably hop in place (equally, injured to uninjured side), skip rope, and/or shadow box comfortably, this more advanced exercise can be helpful to your knee rehab effort.

Jump one-legged bunny hops in four directions (front, back, and to each side). Compare right to left for deficits. As you get better, the hops can be higher and farther in each direction.

FUNCTIONAL DRILLS

There is only so much you can do in the gym, training room, or rehab setting to train your knee for full return to sports and other leisure activities. To prepare yourself for that final phase after knee surgery or rehabilitation, you should work through a variety of functional progressions, including the neuromuscular training outlined earlier in this section. In some instances, a knee brace is a good idea (check with your doctor).

We are now learning that many ACL tears (and re-tears) are preventable with certain year-round conditioning programs. Once you are comfortable jogging straight ahead, you can start some running-and-cutting drills on a field, like a football receiver going out for a pass.

Jog forward in a straight line approximately 10 yards and then, as you continue to jog, slightly angle off either to the right or left as if you were driving a car going off an exit

SKATEBOARD SLIDE

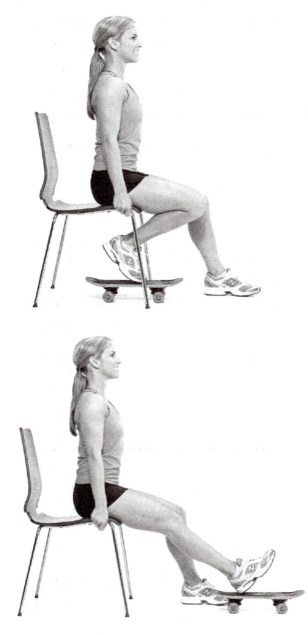

ramp with a gentle curve. (Start with gentle flairs at half speed going to the right and left and progress to faster speeds and sharper curves. You can also "stop on a dime" and do a 90-degree turnout both right and left.) Also, jogging in figure-eight patterns is very helpful. (Start slowly over a 20-yard distance and gradually increase your speed and tighten the figure eight to 10 yards.)

Cartilage Regeneration

We have now entered the era of regenerative (as opposed to reparative) orthopedic surgery, which means that we can sometimes actually regenerate damaged tissue or structures, including joint cushions. We have covered this quite extensively in this book, and it is very exciting for knee surgeons and their patients alike. There are several procedures that can be used to try to regrow injured or damaged knee cushions, and the two that I most commonly perform are microfracture surgery and autologous chondrocyte implantation or transplantation (ACI).

Microfracture surgery, developed by my friend and one of my mentors, Dr. Richard Steadman in Vail, Colorado, is a relatively simple arthroscopic outpatient procedure that counts on your body's own stem cells to patch the damaged area. However, ACI is a more involved open surgery in which your own cartilage cells are actually implanted after having been grown in the laboratory.

In both types of surgery, the recovery is relatively slow and a staged progressive rehabilitation program is critical and every bit as important as the surgery itself. Often, patients have more difficulty with the post-operative restrictions and rehabilitation than the actual surgery. People don't like restrictions placed upon them, especially if they (and their knee) are feeling well, but this is one time when your body can deceive you. You might feel well pretty quickly, but the inside of your knee is not ready for prime time.

It takes tremendous patience, but failure to follow the protocol outlined here can result in suboptimal results. Both surgeries involve a period of approximately 8 to 12 weeks of limited weight bearing, and crutches or a brace, depending on the location of the repaired damage (kneecap versus femoral condyle). For the first 3 or 4 weeks, passive motion of the knee helps regrow the cushion. A CPM (continuous passive motion) machine is often prescribed for 6 to 8 hours per day. For people who don't have a large chunk of time or insurance coverage for CPM, I substitute the "skateboard slide" (see page 167) that I came up with as I talked on the phone and my foot rocked back and forth on my son Dylan's skateboard. (You can get a child-size mini-skateboard for under $5.00 at discount stores, and rocking your leg/knee back and forth can simulate the CPM use.)

More specific rehabilitation programs for microfracture can be found at Dr. Steadman's Web site (www.steadman-hawkins.com). Information about chondrocyte transplantation can be found at www.carticel.com.

The FrameWork Fix: Start with recovery exercises (page 152) and progress to water exercise, the elliptical machine, and strength training when you get the green light from your surgeon. I do not recommend high-impact loading like running or sports for approximately 9 months because the newly formed joint cushion needs adequate time to mature and become more durable. During the knee recovery period you can continue to strengthen your opposite leg and work on your core and upper-extremity strength and flexibility. The full cycle of knee cushion regrowth and maturation can take up to 2 years, so you must be extremely patient. Hopefully we can accelerate this process with the new cell therapies on the horizon.

Knee Stress Fracture

Stress fractures can occur anywhere in the body and are even seen about the knee area, especially in the upper or proximal tibia (more on the medial/inner side) or in the patella. Unlike traumatic fractures that happen from a sudden trauma or injury, stress fractures occur from repetitive microtrauma over time. This is similar to a paperclip that gets bent back and forth. First it is fine, and then it starts to fatigue, and, eventually, if you keep bending it, it will break.

The earliest phase of a stress fracture is called a stress reaction. If you continue to pound on it with activities, cracks can begin to develop and a stress fracture forms. This is a potentially serious situation as the bone can further break or shatter once it is weakened.

Stress fractures are usually a result of overuse without adequate rest and recovery between workouts. There is often a change in workout duration, intensity, or frequency that precipitates these breakdowns, and there may be underlying biomechanical or technical issues. Women are particularly susceptible, and those who overtrain to the point of a dramatic loss in body fat suspend their usual flow of hormones, which leads to loss of bone density (especially if there is inadequate calcium and vitamin D intake), which leads to a significantly higher incidence of stress fractures.

Stress fractures are often not seen on x-rays, especially early in the process. An MRI or bone scan will make the diagnosis in most cases. (I prefer MRI as there is no radiation involved and it is more accurate.) More generally, stress fractures underscore the importance of exercise as a managed dose—too much of a good thing can indeed lead to damage.

The FrameWork Fix: Depending on the type, location, and severity of the stress fracture, your do's and don'ts will vary, but you will in all probability need to stop the activity that caused it until the fracture heals enough to withstand higher forces again. You should be able to remain fit with alternate low-impact workouts, especially in the water or perhaps on a bike or elliptical machine. This is best determined by your treating physician, who hopefully will find a creative way to keep you fit while the fracture heals.

It's important to strengthen the surrounding musculature. If there is an alignment issue, an unloader brace or heel wedge may be helpful. Depending on the sport or fitness activity you participate in, work with a coach or trainer to redesign your program, and consider orthotics. Because so many overuse injuries such as stress fractures are rooted in either faulty techniques or faulty program design, especially consider any sudden change or increase in intensity, duration, or frequency of the activity. For women, evaluate your menstrual cycle and improve the amount of calcium and vitamin D in your diet.

Pre- and Post-Knee Replacement

Knee replacement surgery (total knee arthroplasty, or TKA) is one of the most efficacious surgeries across all surgical disciplines when one considers success rates, patient outcomes, and patient satisfaction. I believe knee replacement patients can enjoy even more success with the right pre- and post-operative exercise routines (see the Joint Discussion on page 184). Unfortunately, many joint replacement surgeons fail to optimize their patients' functional results by not focusing more on exercise and fitness. I think this is beginning to change, but not enough for me.

Many patients with arthritis, especially the elderly, have become very weak and deconditioned because of the pain and inactivity, and I don't just mean their knee or knees. The weakness involves their entire bodies: musculoskeletal structure, cardiovascular system, and metabolism. Many are overweight. Many are in too much pain preoperatively to work on their fitness, but that is where physical therapy, and perhaps a water-based program, can help. The stronger and fitter you are going into the surgery, the quicker and more complete your recovery will be.

The FrameWork Fix: After the surgery, knee rehabilitation and overall fitness are essential. In the early phases, the main goal is to learn to walk again (often with crutches, a walker, or a cane initially), to reduce swelling and pain, and to regain mobility, especially lost motion. This is more difficult and takes more effort if the knee is stiff, with lost motion (extension and/or flexion), before surgery. Physical therapy can help tremendously, especially in the early postoperative period. Once the knee settles down, you can focus on regaining strength and endurance in not only your knee and leg, but also your entire body.

Start with the Knee Range-of-Motion exercises (page 156). Add the skateboard slide (page 167) if needed. Once you have had 90 degrees of flexion, you can try a stationary bike with no resistance. (Remember, motion is lotion.) Also, when your wound is fully healed, you can try water-based exercise like water walking, Knee Range-of-Motion in water, and the use of a kickboard.

Regaining strength is critical. Start with the Lock-and-Lift Isometrics (page 154), "Short Arcs" (page 155), and/or elastic tubing (page 155). Also work on the tree pose discussed on page 184. Hopefully, you will be able to progress to all of the knee exercises, including the hip and core work on pages 134 to 145. What is usually not permitted after TKA is kneeling and/or running, but you can still be in terrific shape and enjoy many lower-impact sports and activities.

BUILT TO LAST

If you've been lucky enough to avoid the Top 10 most common knee ailments and injuries so far, congratulations. Unfortunately, time itself is causing changes in your body that make at least one of them far more likely to become your companion in the future. Again, the FrameWork program is all about extending the warranty on your frame.

If you have difficulty with these or other musculoskeletal ailments, get them checked out earlier rather than later. Often a simple rehabilitation program can get you out of trouble. Better yet, put prevention to work now.

Monitor your body for signs and symptoms of these and other frame-related ailments. Also, perform the self-test regularly so you can nip any potential problems in the bud before they sideline you. The FrameWork program offers plenty of protection from these and most musculoskeletal problems, so that you can count on being more durable for life, with a frame that is solid, and a body that's built to last.

A LEG UP ON AN ACTIVE LIFE

Whether you define "active" as being able to play competitive singles tennis or as being able to move about and perform your usual daily tasks, you'll be "active for life" if you commit to a regular workout program. The specifics and level of your physical fitness are unique to you, but *action* is something that applies to every case.

Hurting or not, your frame requires attention if it is to recover from injury and stay healthy. The whole idea is to do the appropriate targeted exercises (the ones you can tolerate), and progress at your own pace. Remember, this is not a competition.

It sometimes takes a little detective work to determine which exercises are best for your situation, and which should be avoided. Use the ones that work best for you more often and avoid those that cause significant discomfort (but don't forget to try them again later when your knee improves). Over time, and with some trial and error, you will probably develop your own optimal routine, as this is not a one-size-fits-all program.

If you are having difficulty advancing, try adding only one new exercise per session to see how you tolerate it. Sometimes an exercise feels good while you are doing it, but later that evening, or the next day, you are in trouble. If you've added numerous exercises, it's difficult to determine which one or two are the culprits. You might have to stay at a low level of exercise indefinitely, or you might wind up going back and forth between challenge levels, but that's okay. As long as you keep taking steps, however small, your frame will be in far better shape down the road.

"Kneed" More?

The information that follows is for anyone with ongoing knee problems or issues, but it is especially useful for those "tweeners" we mentioned in Step 2 who have a chronic knee condition for which there is no immediate surgical or other cure. They may have even already had surgery (or surgeries), but there's not enough justification for another surgical procedure at this point in time. In other words, these are nonsurgical steps you can take, alone or in combination, that may improve how your knee feels or functions on a day-to-day basis.

Tweeners and other "knee-dy" unfortunates are saddled with limitations, including compromised mobility that is often accompanied by pain and weakness. This sets in motion the vicious cycle, also introduced in Step 2, that spirals ever downward. Quad deterioration shows up within weeks of inactivity, and that leads to higher impact, loading, and other forces across the knee which cause more pain, which leads to a further reduction in activity and even more weakness. More serious damage, such as torn menisci, chondral defects, and ligament sprains, are a fait accompli—unless you intercede and break the cycle.

We've already discussed a lot of weapons in the fight for healthy knees, and we're about to add a few more, but the one constant that should inform all of your efforts to get better is that every step you take is one that leads to maximum activity. Put another way, it is perfectly okay to seek relief from pain, but that is only step one in the recovery process. The main objective should always be gaining the ability to exercise and move more. That, my friend, leads to permanent improvement.

END THE VICIOUS CYCLE

You can go only so far with heat and ice and ibuprofen and naproxen, and many recommendations and treatments from doctors have a shelf life as well. It sure is frustrating to be at the mercy of one's knee or knees, in constant search for improvement. Trust me, as proactive as I am about taking care of mine, there are times when it gets to me, too. It's not outside the realm of possibility that I myself will be seriously considering a total knee replacement at some point, but my real goal is to delay that as long as possible or to avoid it completely. I feel your pain as I pass along what I know about what people with chronic problem hinges can do. First and foremost in this regard is that you won't make much progress if you don't start out with a positive, proactive attitude about finding help. The solution isn't always immediately visible, nor is it always traditional approaches that will get you where you want to go. I've learned to keep a wide-open mind in terms of treatment alternatives.

DON'T FORGET FIRST AID

If the over-the-counter (OTC) products you use have lost their effectiveness, switch to other ones or try something new. Just don't mix NSAIDs. I have many patients who've taken a variety of over-the-counter NSAIDs at the same time. Not only is that dangerous, but no one medication can reach maximum effectiveness if there are others on board. If one is not working for you after a few weeks, it is reasonable to try a different one because there is individual responsiveness to NSAID medications, but always check in with your physician first—especially if you're taking them like M&Ms.

One thing that is safe to use while you're taking NSAIDs is Tylenol, and the combination (at the same time, or at different times during the day) can be helpful for many. In fact, to avoid the many potential problems with NSAIDs, I have personally switched to extra-strength Tylenol as a mainstay around heavier activities, sports, or workouts, and I suggest the same to my active achy patients. I have been impressed with its ability to take the edge off my discomfort and allow me to remain active and fit. Tylenol may also be a better choice because NSAIDs have been shown to have some potential negative implications for optimal musculoskeletal recovery, as they can interfere with bone healing, joint surface regrowth, and tendon repair. The decision to use an NSAID for sports-related injuries should be driven by the need for anti-inflammatory relief, rather than for pain relief alone, and there should be time limits on use, something best determined by your physician and the nature of your injury.

Also, don't be afraid to experiment a little with ice and heat and with new patches, lotions, and balms, such as Voltaren Gel (diclofenac, a topical NSAID), that appear regularly. There is a new topical treatment (Pennsaid) that combines diclofenac with the old pain-relieving standby DMSO (dimethyl sulfoxide), and it is approved for treatment of osteoarthritis of the knee. There is also a diclofenac patch that can be worn all day, marketed as the Flector Patch. Some arthritis patients do pretty well with topical capsaicin (Zostrix cream), a natural pain reliever that, when applied to the skin, reduces and even temporarily depletes levels of Substance P, a pain neurotransmitter. The capsaicin is pepperlike, and it can burn a little and even cause some skin irritation. (A word to the wise: Wash your hands thoroughly after applying it and never get any in your eyes.) All of these types of agents are worth some trial and error because they provide relief for many knees and other joints. (One exception: As much as I am a fan of the joint supplements glucosamine and chondroitin sulfate, I cannot support their use in topical ointments. As I've said before, glucosamine and chondroitin sulfate help many individuals, but you need to find a high-quality brand and take it orally, rather than rub it around your knee.)

YOUR PHYSICIAN AND HCP

There are many different types of doctors and health-care professionals (HCPs) who can help your knees, from your primary physician and/or chiropractor to your orthopedic surgeon, rheumatologist, or primary-care sports medicine specialist. It often takes a "village"— a team approach that includes other HCPs, such as physical therapists (PTs), certified athletic trainers (ATCs), and podiatrists. However, if you are not getting better, you must consult with an orthopedic surgeon who has years of added training and experience with the body's frame and musculoskeletal system. Find one who specializes in the knee, as he or she will be up on the latest and best information. Discuss the modalities here that interest you and get some input. Your specialist may think it's time to inject cortisone or a viscosupplement ("lubricant") such as Synvisc-One, and if it's been a while since your last visit, there just might be something new in the way of stim treatments, scaffolds, grafts, and the like that can be offered to you. Maybe there's a new brace he or she knows about that will do the trick for you. At the very least, your specialist should supervise or assess the care provided by other professionals across multiple disciplines with whom you would like to work.

Chronic knees demand professional attention, but don't necessarily settle for the first doctor or other specialist you meet. You may connect better with the second or third one, or find someone farther outside the box if you're stymied. Sometimes you even need a different kind of second opinion. One thing I've learned from years working with dancers and other high-level professional athletes is that many sports injuries, especially the nagging, chronic, recurrent overuse variety, are rooted not in a single obvious injury, but in technical flaws you bring to the event. I can get most injured dancers better, but often it also takes a consultation with a ballet master skilled in technique to find the subtle, biomechanical bad habit that is the root of the dancer's problem. Ditto for tennis players and their stroke mechanics. Instead of recommending more doctors, more MRIs, or more cortisone shots, I often recommend working with a knowledgeable coach, trainer, or instructor to see why a patient is getting into trouble. There are even centers that specialize in biomechanical analysis of athletes using high-speed computerized video technology. You don't hear a doctor say this often, but in medicine, we don't know everything. Sometimes we have to tap into the knowledge of others.

FLOOR TO CORE

Simple changes to your footwear can make all the difference in some cases. This could involve

JOINT DISCUSSION

I recently gave a keynote speech at a Synvisc national sales meeting. I applaud their efforts and that of other companies to consistently develop new and better products that I use for problem knee joints that allow my patients to stay active.

The topic of my presentation was the downhill spiral of arthritis that results in a vicious cycle of knee woe: Pain leads to lack of use, which leads to weakness and stiffness, which leads to less use, which leads to more serious knee and overall health deterioration.

For the umpteenth time: Motion is lotion. Find someone or something to keep you going.

a change in sneaker type, or the addition of pads, lifts, wedges, or inserts. All of these can affect how your leg and knee work. As I've said before, healthy knees start on the floor (or ground) and end with the core. From a biomechanical standpoint, the knee is tremendously influenced by the foot and ankle. This is especially true of patellar pain syndromes and overuse injuries in runners and dancers. This is why a thorough knee evaluation includes the foot and ankle, hip, and the core in addition to the knee itself. Unequal leg lengths, anatomical alignment issues, and foot/ankle over- or underpronation can often be helped by different types of inserts in shoes or sneaks; some are available over the counter, while others are custom and costly. Check with your orthopedic surgeon and/or podiatrist to see if these simple measures can help you.

IMPROVED LIFESTYLE

Your knee problems will get a whole lot better a whole lot faster if you do everything you can first to help matters. If you're battling a knee problem without being in the best shape you can be in, you're fighting with one hand tied behind your back. Revisit Step 4 on a regular basis: You simply must eat properly, take appropriate high-quality supplements,

de-stress, maintain a healthy weight, stop smoking if that applies, keep alcohol to no more than a glass of red wine per day or three to four cocktails per week in separate sittings, and exercise in whatever way you can.

No surprise that I mention yet again the importance of getting going to keep you going. Time and time again, studies have shown the powerful healing effects of exercise, and a recent one touted tai chi and yoga as effective treatments for knee arthritis and knee pain. If you can't handle rigorous programs, keep working at the Recovery Program and/or easier levels of exercises in the previous step (with a therapist if necessary). It doesn't matter if you can only do the first step of the first routine. That's a start to the next one if you keep at it.

PHYSICAL THERAPY ("KNEEHABILITATION")

You might have discomfort when you exercise, and it can be significant at times, but if you work with your doctor and/or therapist, you'll stay on the safe side of the pain-injury line and reap the wonderful benefits exercise provides. Your physical therapist or certified athletic trainer can guide you through safe, effective routines and help you get through those painful stumbling blocks we all encounter on the road to recovery. He or she can teach you the important difference between hurt and harm and advance your program when you are ready, documenting your progress along the way.

Unfortunately, in these modern times of health-care reform, too many insurers have created financial disincentives for patients in need of physical therapy. Higher co-pays and limited numbers of therapy visits have resulted in patients not getting the full extent and benefits of therapy that they desperately need. This makes it even more important for patients to learn what they must do on their own to maximize their recovery. Health clubs are experiencing an expanding role in this regard, and I have worked with fitness professionals and personal trainers to help make them more knowledgeable in dealing with clients with a variety of musculoskeletal issues. I have collaborated with the American Council on Exercise (ACE) to develop advanced education and certification courses (*Your Client's FrameWork*) targeting this issue. In my mind, health clubs are a natural extension of health-care delivery and to date have been underutilized in this capacity. This whole

KNEEPAD

A recent article revealed again the link between smoking and joint problems, and this particular one connected this very destructive habit with the advanced arthritis that causes knee pain.

area is getting more and more important with our aging population and aging Baby Boomers.

BRACES

You can choose from a wide variety of supports, which fall into two categories—comfort braces or functional braces. Some are better than others for a specific condition, some are of no help, and a couple might actually be contraindicated. Most patients will fit standard off-the-shelf models; some have knees with a very unique size or shape that requires a total custom fit. In these cases, precise measurements are taken so the proper brace can be constructed.

If you've got a chronic knee problem, it is likely that the braces on hooks in the local pharmacy aren't of much use. They might be better than nothing, but don't fall into a habit where you just do what you've always done. Instead, spend some time with someone who has the most up-to-date skills in this area. You just might discover a whole new world, one in which you play a more active part.

Comfort Braces

These are neoprene or elastic bandages that you usually can get in most pharmacies or even some sporting goods stores. They provide minimal if any support but do increase warmth under the brace, which keeps things loose enough for exercise and thus improves your overall comfort. They also can help to improve proprioception (you're comfortable with this word by now, aren't you?). Maybe they just serve as a reminder for you not to overdo it or abuse your knee.

I am always asked by patients whether these knee supports will mask pain and potentially cause more damage, or if one can get "addicted" to using them, and I can reassure you that they are very safe to use and there is no harm in trying them. I like the ones that are more of a wrap, with Velcro for easy on and off, rather than the pull-on ones that are sometimes difficult to get on and off, especially in warmer weather and when you have been sweating.

Some individuals feel better if there is some support or there are some hinges on the medial and lateral side. If you have kneecap arthritis or patellofemoral pain syndrome (PFPS), you should use the style with a hole cut out for the kneecap (which I also suggest for most other knee issues). Some even have a buttress to help support the kneecap.

There are some more sophisticated patellar braces (for example, a Palumbo or Shields brace) made specifically for individuals who have loose kneecaps and tend to sublux or dislocate them. They're designed to dynamically keep your kneecap in place by tightening certain straps and having certain pads in certain places. Also, a group of researchers from Belgium studying individuals with patellar pain had them do flexion and extension knee exercises while the researchers recorded brain activity with functional MRIs. They found that wearing the brace not only helped proprioception around the knee itself, but also resulted in change of brain activity, suggesting that there may actually be a higher neural effect when a brace is worn.

Functional Braces

Earlier versions were constructed with materials that made them a bit cumbersome and a bit scary, but they're now made of such lightweight materials that they can be comfortably worn while you're playing sports.

We even have a brace now for those with arthritis and alignment issues. It's called an un-loader brace because it actually shifts knee alignment like surgical removal of bone does. Individuals who are knock-kneed or bowlegged and have arthritis in one compartment can sometimes have the pressure taken off the worn, painful side of their knee and be more comfortable with everyday activities and sports. Some newer knee braces incorporate pulsed electromagnetic waves to help reduce pain and inflammation and promote cartilage regrowth and regeneration, something that clearly needs more research. One of my mentors, Dr. Carl Brighton, a brilliant researcher, helped develop this technology

that shows promise for wounded knees. It should not be confused with magnets placed in knee sleeves or braces, which have never been scientifically proven to do anything.

Some patients with knee instability, who are candidates for surgical tightening of ligaments such as the ACL, opt just to use a custom brace instead. Same for folks with a torn PCL. With the right fit, a brace can often keep your knee from going out on you, and it can stabilize a sprained PCL or other soft tissue enough to give the knee every chance to improve on its own. Even those who have had surgery for a torn ACL or other major ligament injury will

KNEEPAD

Options for Filling Your "Kneeds"

- First aid
- See your doctor
- Check and recheck Step 4
- Physical therapy
- Braces
- Acupuncture
- Other knee modalities

JOINT DISCUSSION

Years ago, I spent a month in China on a medical exchange program. It was one of the first of its kind as China was trying to enter the era of modern medicine. We taught the Chinese practitioners much of our sports medicine advancements, and we experienced firsthand many traditional Eastern interventions, including acupuncture. The experience was tremendous; I was quite impressed with the results I witnessed, and my mind was opened forever. More recently, functional MRI (fMRI) studies have documented reproducible changes in brain activity when acupuncture needles are inserted.

find a friend in a quality brace, although the final verdict is not in as to whether everyone really needs a brace to go back to sports after a ligament reconstruction. This is best determined by your surgeon. I prefer that my patients wear an ACL brace for the first 6 to 12 months of playing sports again.

ACUPUNCTURE

I think it's safe to say that most people steer away from any optional procedure that involves needles. If you're stymied by your knee, however, it wouldn't hurt to get a consultation with a highly respected acupuncturist. Studies with patients who had arthritis have shown significant improvement for those who underwent this treatment, and the long-term follow-up showed that treated patients continued to improve. If nothing else is working for you, this might be worth a look.

OTHER KNEE MODALITIES

There are more and more modalities that can help reduce knee pain and ultimately improve function. Ultrasound and electrical stimulation can be used for a variety of knee conditions. Corticosteroid creams or other pain-reducing gels can be used in conjunction with ultrasound or electrical stimulation. Phonophoresis and iontophoresis techniques can help drive those molecules to deeper tissues to reduce pain and inflammation, as well as enhance healing at deeper tissue levels.

JOINT DISCUSSION

During my surgical training, I had the opportunity to work at a hospital where one of the anesthesiologists was trained in the use of acupuncture. (This was way before its use became popular in the United States. In fact, the entire field of "alternative medicine" had yet to emerge.) The anesthesiologist's daughter had a torn meniscus that needed surgery, and back then there was no arthroscopic surgery, so the old-fashioned open, deep cut–type procedure was laid on.

The anesthesiologist wanted to use acupuncture instead of a traditional general anesthetic. This meant that the patient would be wide awake with a variety of acupuncture needles placed around her face, arms, and chest area. Of course, we were reluctant, but we agreed to give it a try with the proviso that we could give a general anesthetic right away if she experienced any pain.

She had the entire open procedure with acupuncture only. She had no pain whatsoever and talked throughout the procedure. Interestingly, she often would pull her leg toward herself. She was unaware of this, and would stop when we asked her. This reflex movement was really a pain withdrawal response. So her leg and nervous system knew that something painful was happening, but she was not consciously experiencing it. The surgery went fine, and she recovered fully and comfortably. Pretty amazing, wouldn't you say? Another mind opener.

Muscle Stimulation

This not only enhances recovery, it prevents muscle loss and atrophy around injuries, which is why it's been used to treat a variety of sports injuries. It's the perfect way for those who are in too much pain or too weak to exercise to start rebuilding strength after injury, surgery, or immobilization.

H-Wave (Electronic Waveform Lab) is a terrific electrical stimulation device with a unique waveform. It not only reduces the pain of acute and chronic injuries but is terrific for nerve-related pain. (It is theorized that it enhances healing through changes in micro circulation and nitric oxide concentration at the tissue level.) With acute injuries, it can reduce swelling and inflammation, which results in pain reduction and quicker recovery.

H-Wave has also been shown to expedite muscle recovery after vigorous workouts. Only available in the clinical setting at one time, it is now available in the form of a home unit. Newer devices like the InterX neurostimulator (Neuro Resource Group) provide a unique targeted interactive neural stimulation that I believe works on acupuncture-type principles.

JOINT DISCUSSION

Prolotherapy (and Other Things I DON'T Like)

Prolotherapy involves the injection (usually multiple) of an irritant solution into the soft tissues around the knee and other joints. The theory is that scar tissue forms, and possibly a "healing" response occurs, resulting in improved stability and less pain for a variety of chronic knee problems. This treatment modality has become popular in some circles (usually not with orthopedic surgeons). I do not recommend it. I have not seen any convincing controlled scientific data to warrant this invasive intervention, and I believe that the limited success seen with it can be attributed primarily to the placebo effect. I have seen way too many children with elusive patellar pain syndromes exposed to this treatment.

As with prolotherapy, there are other things being injected into knees with claims they can "regrow" articular cartilage or joint cushions. There are ads (especially in airplane magazines) showing pre- and post-injection x-rays with knee joint space and cushioning improved after injection therapy. Please don't be fooled by this. These treatments are costly and not typically covered by insurance. Although there is some promising research in this very area (see the Afterword), we do not yet have a substance that, when injected, will reform or regrow your joint cushion. If it looks too good to be true (and if they're asking for cash up front), it probably is.

As mentioned previously, simple magnets placed around any joints, including your knee, have never been shown to do any more than a placebo. They are still very useful, however, for keeping things on your refrigerator.

JOINT DISCUSSION

I can't tell you how many times patients brought me x-rays that pass with flying colors after a surgical procedure and told me their mobility was okay but that something just didn't feel quite right. More regularly than I prefer, a specific exercise or a specific program was the key missing ingredient. A particular story in this vein comes to mind.

I got to know a woman at my gym after we bumped into each other a few times, and when she told me she needed a total knee replacement, I referred her to a top-notch guy. I didn't see her for about 9 months after the procedure and was thrilled when I ran into her again. (She was smart enough to go back to the health club; some people aren't and/or their doctors discourage them.) I seized the opportunity to catch up with her and talk about my favorite subject.

"I'm lifting weights and doing okay," she said, in a way a lot of patients do. "But something just doesn't feel right."

I knew the procedure had been done correctly, and I could see that she was doing everything in her power to help things along. I also knew that full recovery usually takes a year. Medical detective that I am, however, I couldn't resist a simple biomechanical investigation to see if something had been missed.

"Try the yoga tree pose on your good leg," I said to her. She did quite well with her eyes both open and closed.

I then asked her to do the same on her surgically repaired leg. She couldn't even get into position, let alone hold it for any length of time, even with her eyes wide open. That sure was an "eye-opener" for her.

She had had major surgery, with new parts installed, and no matter how careful the surgeon is, some nerves are cut and they take a long time—and a lot of prodding—to come back. It was apparent to me that she hadn't regained the necessary proprioception in her new knee joint. It's like getting a brand-new computer, with all the bells and whistles, but you still have dial-up connectivity and not high-speed access. I was thrilled again to offer her some simple advice that could really make a difference in how her new knee worked for her, how she *functioned.*

"Hold on to something lightly with one or two fingers until you can balance without holding on," I continued, "and then start just trying to do the yoga tree pose with your eyes open. Build up to where your eyes are closed and you don't need to hold on to anything. After that, just get better and better at it."

A month or so later, she told me it was like night and day for her. Needless to say, that was what I was most thrilled about.

This simple handheld device, which is being seen in more and more training rooms and on sidelines on game day more often, helps manage both acute and chronic pain.

Shock Wave Therapy and Ablation

Chronic knee pain can be caused by tendinitis or tendinopathy (more chronically damaged tendon), and any chronically inflamed tendon is fair game for this "shocking" approach. Extra Corporeal Shock Wave Therapy (ECSWT) uses a spark plug to generate shock waves that disrupt scar tissue, similar to lithotripsy that is used to noninvasively break up and treat kidney stones. By causing microscopic damage to that tissue, new blood vessel formation is induced in the injured areas, facilitating the healing process.

Another new intervention for chronic jumper's knee uses radio waves (coblation microtenotomy) to promote the growth of blood vessels in and around damaged tendons. This minimally invasive surgical procedure uses the Topaz device (a small, handheld wand) to repair areas of tendon damage and avoid larger surgical procedures. These technologies are now being applied to other common ailments, including tennis or golf elbow and heel pain.

ACTIVE FOR LIFE

Even if you have been around the block with several specialists and haven't been helped much, keep going back because news breaks all the time and something just published or new to the market might be the trick you need.

Sometimes it's just a simple thing that can make a world of difference. Everything should be in play so that you can play more. If you have the right brace that unloads your knee, you will move better. If you get a Synvisc injection, you'll have some added lubrication to keep friction down in your knee so you can move better. H-Wave, acupuncture, stim—they all help to one degree or another in getting you on the go. When you move your knees better, you're more active—even if that just means walking better.

Remember: Active is what it is all about, even if it's only at a recovery level. Cortisone isn't a silver bullet; you can't just "inject and go" and not think about your knee until the pain really flares up again. As a rule, an injection is a golden opportunity to participate in your own recovery. It is the first step in a series that *you* must complete. It's designed to temporarily reduce pain while your knee and you start the real work.

Knee exercise is critical for breaking the vicious cycle regardless of the shape you're in. If you want to overcome a balky knee, just get going and do the things you can do to improve your frame's hinges. Some of my patients take a long time before they come around to the simple fact that, when it comes to knee health, they're a huge part of the solution. There is only so much your physician can do. If they can help break the vicious cycle, then the rest is up to you. Lifestyle changes likely need to be effected along with the regular exercise that plays as important a role as the most talented physician. (When choosing doctors, make sure you work only with those who recognize the importance of exercise and biomechanical training in your recovery.)

If you don't buy into exercise and don't do your frame work, chances are the doctors you look up and everything they try will be far less effective than they could be.

AFTERWORD

If a doctor is doing his or her job the right way, keeping up with the latest advances is much more than a sometime thing. My world is always evolving. When I'm between cases in the surgery suite (a huge chunk of my life), in the back of my mind I'm thinking about a research paper I just read or how the procedure I'm doing might be improved, all to better help my patients.

As I indicated in Step 2, I think the focus in the future will be on enhancing and accelerating the healing process. The future won't just be about *reparative* medicine, either—it'll be about *regenerative* medicine. It won't be a matter of patching an injury or fixing it up the best we can; it'll be how you get back to the stuff you had originally.

I can hardly wait to use the things discussed below that are in the foreseeable future for our trusty old hinges. And, truth be told, if you are doing your frame work the right way, you'll keep an eye out for them, too.

THE CUTTING EDGE

There's a whole lot of fun stuff going on in the OR with the latest techno toys. At the top of the list is the Minimally Invasive Surgery (MIS) discussed in Step 2. We surgeons are always looking to make incisions smaller so that pain is minimized and the recovery is faster.

Major progress in procedures and equipment, and in the development of artificial parts, seems to occur almost daily in one place or another. Image resolution and surgical instruments get better all the time. Robots and remote procedures (in which the surgeon controls the operation from the city where he or she practices) are getting closer every day. Computer navigation is being used in many ORs to allow for more precise joint replacement and ligament reconstruction placement.

STEM CELLS AND BMPS

The broadest front in the movement toward regenerative medicine is stem-cell research.

Stem cells are structures that have not yet differentiated into skin cells, muscle cells, soft tissue cells, or other types of cells. This means that they still have the potential to become almost anything. By manipulating stem cells in the right way, biomedical researchers can use them as a sort of universal building material, cultivating just about any tissue or spare part needed.

At a company called Osiris Therapeutics in Baltimore, scientists extracted stem cells from goat bone marrow and allowed them to multiply in a glass dish. Then they injected 10 million of these cells into the arthritic knees of goats, and the tissues that had worn away began to grow back. The new cells also slowed the rate of joint erosion, meaning stem cell therapy holds the promise of prevention as well as repair. This would be true disease modification, rather than our current approach of just treating symptoms.

The same principle applies to the therapeutic use of naturally occurring substances called bone morphogenic proteins (BMPs), which are produced on various occasions throughout our lives. They "turn on" for the first time before birth, when they spur growth in the fetus. They also turn on whenever we are in a growth stage or break a bone. Most tissues heal with a scar that is different from what was there before; however, the healing tissue in bone, largely because of the action of BMPs, is identical to what was there before. Ideally, we want other tissue to have this capacity to perfectly replicate itself, in its original format, in the healing process, rather than forming scar tissue only.

Scientists have now developed a genetically engineered form of BMP that's been approved by the U.S. Food and Drug Administration. These proteins induce bone formation and enhance fracture repair, and can be used as an alternative for bone grafts in healing difficult fractures and in spinal fusion surgery. This means you don't have to "borrow" bone from somewhere else in your body because BMPs basically come in a jar off a shelf. We know there are a few BMPs that have the potential to form articular cartilage and thus reform damaged joint cushions. Hopefully, we'll have the same for tendons, ligaments, and menisci. The impact is going to be tremendous, with wide applicability in the treatment of a variety of frame issues.

OTHER CELL TECHNOLOGIES

A platelet-rich plasma (PRP) injection was referenced in Step 1, and it and similar technologies to "juice up" recovery from ACL reconstructions and other surgeries are being perfected. *Accelerated healing* is the term, and the goal is to have grafts incorporate in tunnels faster and become stronger quicker. It's been done in a lab setting with animals and is just hitting ORs around the country, but more research is needed to understand the optimal ways in which these technologies can be used to enhance these and other surgical procedures.

We're also making strides with those rebuilding "scaffolds" introduced in Step 2 (for meniscus reconstruction instead of removal) to repair torn ACLs. New scaffold formulations are being concocted in "mad scientist" labs from various biomaterials to regenerate a variety of frame parts.

As for articular cartilage, the autologous chondrocyte implantation (ACI) procedure, also discussed in Step 2, has been taken to the next level by impregnating the cultured chondrocytes (cartilage cells) into a bioabsorbable collagen scaffold (called Matrix-Induced Autologous Chondrocyte Implantation, or MACI) or patch that can be implanted into the knee through those smaller incisions or even via arthroscopic techniques. There are also techniques that attempt to grow a better line of specialized articular cartilage cells with more of the normal joint surface type II collagen, rather than the type I collagen that sometimes forms that is less durable. I believe this will soon lead to repaving the entire road, which is what is needed to fix truly arthritic, diffusely worn knees, rather than only repairing focal areas of damage. (You can learn more about ACI by visiting www.carticel.com.)

As a "cutting-edge" knee surgeon, I have been very disappointed in our FDA in this very area. They have made it close to impossible for biotechnology companies to bring many of these scaffold technologies, which are widely available now in Europe and other countries, to our patients in the United States. I hope this changes soon, as many patients could benefit from these advancements. Regrettably, the ACI procedure here is still a pretty big, open surgery.

Some knee surgeons, including me, have used a version of the patch that is now available in the United States to make the procedure a little easier on the patient. We use a porcine-based Bio-Gide scaffold (Osteo-Health) to patch the defect in the knee, rather than making a separate incision to obtain the patient's own periosteum (paper-thin tissue covering bone) to cover the defect in the knee joint (like a blowout patch on a tire). This patch has not been approved yet by the FDA for use in the knee, but it is FDA-approved for other surgical purposes, so it is available for use "off-label" in the United States. Bio-Gide has been helpful for those patients who are willing to let us use it. Unfortunately, the FDA has not allowed the cells to be grown directly on the scaffold as is done in Europe. Hopefully, that will soon be the case here.

DESIGNER "GENES" AND "GELS"

An early report from the University of Pittsburgh suggests that recovery from sports-related injuries involving slow-healing tissues can be significantly sped up with gene therapy that enhances growth factors. Someday in the not too distant future, treatments for injured tendons, cartilage, or ligaments will be injections instead of surgical repairs. Your own tissue will be regenerated—like a salamander regrowing its tail.

A bioengineering researcher at the University of Colorado is working on a method whereby damaged areas of articular cartilage can be fixed in a simple matter, almost like spackling a crack or ding in your wall before painting. This technique (not yet ready for humans) uses hydrogel technology, which involves a liquid plastic mixed with TGF-beta (a protein that makes cartilage grow). The combination is injected into the damaged area, after which a tiny fiber-optic light is shined on the material to convert it into a gelatin soft solid. In the weeks to follow, the TGF-beta triggers the growth of new articular cartilage and the plastic part slowly decomposes, leaving behind a new joint surface. Hopefully, these hydrogels will be available for human use soon because they can be mixed with a variety of growth factors to repair and regenerate other body parts.

Other researchers at Northwestern University are using nanotechnology for cartilage regeneration. They employ synthetic bioactive biomaterials, gels, and growth factors (transforming growth factor beta-1) to promote cartilage regeneration.

The logical extension of regenerative medicine is the actual genetic reprogramming of cells. More and more evidence is being uncovered that shows aging is a programmed biological function and not just the inevitable result of simple wear and tear. Although some dedicated people make strides every day, I suspect it will be a while before we can influence the code for breakdown on a microcellular level. In the meantime, the FrameWork program will keep the wear-and-tear part of the equation to a minimum.

CHONDROPROTECTION

Chondroprotection is a big word, but an important one when it comes to the many joints in your body, especially your knees. You may recall that your joint cushions are made of articular cartilage filled with cells called chondrocytes. When your joint cushion is injured, damaged, or grows old, the chondrocytes begin to fail and die. Once this process begins, it can propagate across the joint surface pretty rapidly, leading to arthritis. The great majority of our current pharmaceutical treatments for arthritis (such as NSAIDs) basically just manage the symptoms and really do little or nothing to halt the process and/or protect the chondrocytes (i.e., chondroprotection) from further damage. You may feel better, but the damage often continues to worsen with time.

For years, researchers have been working to develop chondroprotective agents that can actually change or modify the course of the disease process, so that when a joint surface is injured, or if early arthritis is diagnosed, that agent can be given to halt the process in its stride. Chondrocytes, like brain cells, are not replaced or regenerated once they die or are significantly damaged. Several developments have shown promise along this line. Joint supplements such as glucosamine, chondroitin sulfate, and ASU (avocado soy unsaponifiables) have shown promise in tissue culture and in animal and human studies in terms of protecting joint cushions and slowing down the progression of osteoarthritis. It is no wonder that I take Cosamin ASU and recommend it to my patients who have osteoarthritis and those who have had any cartilage regeneration type of surgery such as microfracture or chondrocyte transplantation. There has also been progress in developing substances that can be injected directly into the joint that would not only relieve symptoms but also protect the cushion. Recently presented research using high-tech qualitative MRI has shown that Synvisc-One may have chondroprotective capabilities. This development could be significant and result in viscosupplements being injected much sooner, rather than later, in injured or arthritic joints. Clearly more research is needed in this area, but I can tell you without hesitation, be it a pill, a supplement, or an injection, anything that can prove itself as a chondroprotective agent would be a game changer.

PARTS DEPARTMENT

One of the main goals of the FrameWork program is to prevent the need for knee joint replacement. However, there are times, despite all the best efforts and intentions, that a new knee is your only option to stop the pain and keep you going. The good news, mentioned earlier, is that it is difficult to find another surgical procedure, across all surgical disciplines, that enjoys the extremely high success rates and high patient satisfaction rates that total knee replacement surgery (TKA) has.

As I have mentioned previously, there is an exponential increase in the amount of knee replacements being done, and we are seeing them in younger and younger patients. It is projected that by the year 2016 more than 1 million TKAs will be needed annually in the United States, and this will increase 600 percent to more than 3.4 million knee replacements annually by 2030. Unfortunately, knee replacements don't always last forever. Approximately 95 percent will hold up for about 15 years; at that point, or for the unlucky 5 percent that fail prior to that, revision surgery is necessary. Revisions are a more complex procedure, so it's not as simple as just switching parts and sending you on your way, and there is concern in the orthopedic community that

there may not be enough highly trained joint replacement surgeons to handle the load of primary and revision surgeries. On the plus side, there have been tremendous advancements in the world of knee replacement surgery, and both materials and surgeons (i.e., parts and labor) are getting better every day. Implants are lasting longer, especially if you take good care of them.

In some patients, arthritic damage is isolated to one section or compartment of the knee, and the remainder of the knee is healthy. For them, if they meet certain requirements (age, alignment, and weight), unicompartmental or partial knee replacement is an option.

One gripe I have with many knee replacement surgeons that nags me is a missing exercise and fitness prescription after patients are up and going with their new knees. Studies have shown that patients and surgeons are not always aligned when it comes to expectations, outcomes, and results after joint replacement surgery. I firmly believe that the essential missing ingredient is an exercise and fitness component. I believe that patients will never have the best possible outcome—maximum function—if they remain unfit.

A properly designed exercise program—*FrameWork for the Knee*—is the answer. Push your surgeon to work with you in this regard. You may be opening your surgeon's mind in a way that will help many of his or her future patients.

YOUR PART IN THE FUTURE

Gadgets and gizmos are always improving the knee procedures I do, and the focus on regenerative medicine that is in its infancy will make a lot of them unnecessary someday. But no matter how good things get in the OR, they will still be second best to the original equipment you were born with—your body.

And your body was designed to *move*. Thomas Cureton, an exercise physiologist, wisely noted that "the human body is the only machine that breaks down when not used." He's absolutely right about that. With remarkable advances just around the corner for saving knee parts that aren't too far gone, there's never been a greater incentive to hang on to what you have through proper exercise, nutrition, and some simple lifestyle changes—a framework for the best of health.

ADDITIONAL RESOURCES

WEB SITES

www.aaos.org (American Academy of Orthopaedic Surgeons, or AAOS)

www.ACAtoday.org (the American Chiropractic Association)

www.acefitness.org (American Council on Exercise)

www.aclprevent.com (Santa Monica Orthopaedic and Sports Medicine Group)

www.apta.org (American Physical Therapy Association)

www.carticel.com (Genzyme Corporation)

www.DrNick.com (Dr. Nicholas DiNubile)

www.DrWeil.com (Dr. Andrew Weil, Alternative Medicine)

www.kneeguru.co.uk

www.knee1.com

www.kneepaininfo.com

www.KneeRx.com (Dr. Nicholas DiNubile)

www.kneesociety.org (The Knee Society, focus on joint replacement)

www.nata.org (National Athletic Trainers' Association)

www.nih.gov (National Institutes of Health)

www.orthoinfo.aaos.org (Your Orthopaedic Connection-AAOS consumer site)

www.physsportsmed.com (The Physician and Sportsmedicine)

www.sportsmed.org (The American Orthopaedic Society for Sports Medicine, or AOSSM)

BOOKS

Clinical Orthopaedic Rehabilitation by S. Brent Brotzman, MD, and Kevin E. Wilk, PT, DPT (Mosby, 2003)

FrameWork: Your 7-Step Program for Healthy Muscles, Bones, and Joints by Nicholas A. DiNubile, MD, with William Patrick (Rodale Inc., 2005)

FrameWork for the Lower Back by Nicholas A. DiNubile, MD, with Bruce Scali (Rodale Inc., second edition, 2010)

Insall and Scott Surgery of the Knee by W. Norman Scott (Churchill Livingstone, fourth edition, 2005)

Stretching, 20th Anniversary Revised Edition by Bob Anderson and Jean Anderson (Shelter Publications, 2000)

DVDS

ACL Prevention Program (PEP Program) by Santa Monica Orthopaedic and Sports Medicine Research Foundation (aclprevent .com)

Your Body's FrameWork, with Dr. Nicholas A. DiNubile, as seen originally on PBS (Santa Fe Productions, Inc.)

Your Body's FrameWork Home WorkOut by Nicholas A. DiNubile, MD (Santa Fe Productions, Inc.)

Your Client's FrameWork (for fitness professionals and personal trainers) by Nicholas A. DiNubile, MD (American Council on Exercise—www.acefitness .org)

PRODUCTS

H-Wave.com (neuromuscular stimulation)

Nautilus Freedom Trainer (www.Nautilus.com)

NRG-unlimited.com (InterX nerve stimulator)

Nutramax Labs (www .nutramax.com) (joint supplements)

SPRI Home Knee Fitness products (www.SPRI.com)

- Interchangeable tubing system
- Interchangeable tubing system attachments (interchangeable handle and/or dual handle strap; ankle attachment)
- Stability balls (Xercise balls)
- Xergym door attachment
- Xertube
- Bosu trainer

ACKNOWLEDGMENTS

It is almost impossible to acknowledge the many individuals who have helped influence and shape my thoughts and philosophy as expressed in *FrameWork for the Knee*. Teachers, medical colleagues, patients, and friends, in the gym or on the field, have all had an impact for which I am grateful.

I would also like to extend my sincere gratitude to the following individuals: Arnold Schwarzenegger for his friendship and inspiration over the years and also "the gang" at Oak Productions, especially Lynn Marks; David Caruso, my friend and partner in creating innovative health solutions through technology; Lois de la Haba, my agent, who believed in me and this project from the very beginning; Bruce Scali for his talent, professionalism, and collaboration; the top-notch, enthusiastic team at Rodale, including Karen Rinaldi, John Atwood, Chris Krogermeier, Zach Greenwald, Chris Gaugler, Stephanie Knapp, Mitch Mandel, and Adrienne Bearden-Gardner; Lindsay Messina and Joe Kelly, whose images grace the pages of this book; Roger Schwab for his friendship and thought-provoking discussions and state-of-the-art workouts and facility at Main Line Health and Fitness; Dean Spragia at Nautilus; the Philadelphia 76ers and Pennsylvania Ballet, two first-class organizations I've had the pleasure to work with over the years and where I have learned firsthand the extraordinary capabilities of the human body and that given the right circumstances, healing can indeed be accelerated; Frank Nein for his help and support in cyberspace, especially at www .DrNick.com; the many physicians and health-care professionals who contributed their thoughts, philosophy, and expertise found within the pages of this book, especially my knee mentors, Drs. Paul Lotke, Joe Torg, Jim Nixon, John Joyce, and Richard Steadman; my dedicated staff, Mary Moran and Barb DeJesse; and most importantly, my loving, supportive family—Marybeth, my wife and creative advisor, and my children, Emily and Dylan, who inspire me every single day.

ABOUT THE AUTHORS

NICHOLAS A. DiNUBILE, MD, an orthopedic surgeon specializing in sports medicine and a best-selling author, has served as orthopedic consultant to the Philadelphia 76ers and the Pennsylvania Ballet. His advice has been featured on prime-time television and in the *New York Times,* the *Wall Street Journal,* the *Washington Post,* and *Newsweek.* His award-winning television special, *Your Body's FrameWork,* has been aired on PBS nationwide. Learn more about Dr. DiNubile at DrNick.com.

BRUCE SCALI writes across multiple genres and transforms complex subject matter to make it accessible to every reader.

INDEX

Boldface page references indicate photographs. <u>Underscored</u> references indicate boxed text.